Aid in Dying

The Ultimate Argument

THE CLEAR ETHICAL CASE FOR PHYSICIAN ASSISTED DEATH

Byron Chell

ISBN-13: 9781497374935

ISBN-10: 1497374936

Library of Congress Control Number: 2014908536

CreateSpace Independent Publishing Platform

North Charleston, South Carolina

"We've all got a lot of dying ahead of us. We might as well learn how to go about it."

- Ken Kesey

In 1984 and upon the unexpected death of his son, Ken Kesey wrote an extraordinary letter to his close friends. In later publishing the letter to the world he noted:

"I sincerely hope that I do not — as Richard II worries — 'play the wanton with our woes,' by this display of my family's private grief and publication of my personal correspondence. I mean it only to suggest a path for others wandering in similar pain. We've all got a lot of dying ahead of us. We might as well learn how to go about it."

Death is the natural end of life. There is truly a lot of dying ahead for all of us. We are well advised to learn how to go about it.

Here we discuss one rare choice on the similar path we all wander.

Contents

Preface   ix

Part 1   Introduction   1

    A.   What is "Aid in Dying?"   1

    B.   Very Few Individuals   3

    C.   Is Aid In Dying "Suicide?"   4

    D.   Current Legal Status in the United States   8

    E.   The Legislative Solution   9

    F.   The Ultimate Question   10

    G.   There Are Only Three Categories of Objections   10

    H.   Is Death the Worst Thing That Can Happen To Us?   11

Part 2   Is It Wrong to Hasten Death?   12

    A.   Feelings and Beliefs   12

    B.   A Secular, Pluralistic Society   16

    C.   Can Ethical Inquiry Resolve the Issue?   17

    D.   Ethical Theories, Principles and Values   19

    E.   The Limits of Ethical Inquiry   25

    F.   Diversity, Uncertainty, Freedom, Peace, Toleration 27

Part 3   Is It Wrong for a Physician to Assist?   29

    A.   Historic Moral Distinctions Do Not Apply   30

        1.   Acting to Cause Death or Allowing to Die?   30

        2.   Intent To Relieve Suffering or Cause Death?   32

    B.   Is Aid In Dying Contrary to the Goals of Medicine? 33

    C.   An Exception to the Goals of Medicine   41

    D.   Physician Objection is Permitted   42

    E.   Do We Need Physicians To Participate?   42

    F.   The Physician's Position   43

Part 4   **Will Aid In Dying Cause More Harm Than Good?**   45

A.   "Consequence" Arguments Are Not Arguments Against Aid In Dying Itself   46

B.   Aid in Dying Cannot be Properly Managed and Policed   47

   1.   Coercion   47

   2.   Depressed or Suicidal Persons   53

   3.   Medical Mistakes   55

   4.   Eliminate the Pain   56

   5.   Not Sufficient Suffering   57

   6.   Harm to Families   58

   7.   Harm to the Physician/Patient Relationship   58

   8.   Aid in Dying Cannot Be Limited   59

   9.   What if the Speculated Harms Do Occur?   60

   10.   Speculated Harm versus Known Benefits   61

C.   Slippery Slopes and the "Culture of Death"   62

   1.   Duty to Die   64

   2.   Aid in Dying As Protection   67

   3.   The Fears Are Misdirected   69

   4.   What is the Experience?   74

   5.   Attack the Experience and the Proponents   75

Part 5   **What Aid In Dying is Really About**   76

Part 6   **The Ultimate Conclusion**   80

About the Author   83

Preface

This is for those who live in states where aid in dying is prohibited. This is for those who want help understanding the ethical arguments surrounding physician assisted death. This is especially for those who continue to argue for the criminalization of aid in dying.

Here is the ethical reasoning in support of this end of life choice. All of the traditional and continuing objections are examined. While it is a comprehensive explanation of the ethical arguments, it is not difficult to understand. It will have value to anyone attempting in good faith to follow the debates.

Here it is clearly shown that there are no ethical arguments sufficient to justify the criminalization of aid in dying in the United States. None.

For decades opinion polls have shown a significant majority of Americans support the legal option of aid in dying. With significant majorities in support, why is it yet prohibited in most states?

First, in most of the United States it has historically been a crime to aid or encourage a suicide. The action of the physician in prescribing lethal drugs, even at the request of a competent, terminally ill patient, has been considered aiding a suicide. Second, powerful opponents have fought to maintain assisted death as a crime. In states where public initiative or legislation is attempted, substantial time, energy and funds are expended by some religious organizations and others to continue the criminalization of aid in dying. It is reasonable to expect such opposition to continue.

In the past thirty years much has been written about aid in dying. Books have argued the need for this final option and described in heart-wrenching detail the difficult experiences of dying patients and their families. "How-to" books have been published showing how the dying might go about killing themselves. Many have discussed and expressed opinions of Dr. Kervorkian. There have been detailed histories of euthanasia tracing human thought from ancient to modern times. At this point it is not necessary to further describe the need for or add to those historical commentaries.

Here is the clearest argument for permitting aid in dying. It seeks to be simple but compelling. It confronts all of the reasons for prohibiting aid in dying whether they come from feelings, beliefs, ethical analysis or fears for the future. We address (1) the decision of the dying individual, (2) the role of the physician, and (3) the feared consequences of permitting aid in dying. It is the ultimate argument because, if these considerations do not demonstrate that aid in dying should be permitted, it cannot be established that aid in dying should be permitted.

It is understandable. It is not difficult to grasp what needs to be known to participate in the public debate. But it is hard for most persons to know where to begin. Complicated and confusing feelings, beliefs, ethical and moral issues surround the subject.

This analysis is intended to help you sort through and make sense of the multiple claims that continue to be made regarding aid in dying. You should be able to take any issue, objection or argument you encounter and point to the portion of this explanation where it is addressed. In doing so you can place the argument in context and understand what is meant and why it is or is not valid to the ultimate question.

It is limited. There are hundreds of articles and books addressing this issue written by experts in ethics and mostly read by other experts. Writings in theology, moral and ethical theory, medical tradition, profes-sional roles, legal theory, human psychology and more all analyze the issue and take positions. A complete discussion of those subjects and the arguments for and against aid in dying could cover a ten volume set. But those volumes would be useless to the average person. Here we limit the discussion on every issue with the intent only to reach a point on the road where we can find our way and justify the conclusions.

Because so much has been written one could include hundreds of footnotes, references and citations. The choice has been to exclude them. Either the analysis makes sense and stands on its own or it does not. No authorities are required. The average reader will pay little attention and the expert does not need them.

While there is much wonderful literature on these subjects, anyone who wishes further information relating to any issue can, in this wonderful electronic age, find innumerable sources and materials at the fingertip. It is difficult to appreciate the amount of material available to us in our homes and internet cafes. For any issue, simply search (Google) a word, a phrase or a subject. Be prepared, however, to find yourself on the never-ending roadway of viewpoints that could take months if not years to travel.

Finally, there is no attempt here to change your religious beliefs or your feelings concerning dying and death. There is no attempt to convince physicians that they should accede to the requests of patients to hasten death. Those are matters of individual conscious. Here we focus on aid in dying and public policy.

Part One

Introduction

A. What is "Aid in Dying?"

What do we mean by "aid in dying?" If you are discussing this subject with others, the first rule is to make certain you are discussing the same thing.

What is the proper term to use? Shall we label it "aid in dying?" Shall we call it "physician assisted death" or "physician assisted suicide?" Should we use an acronym such as AID, PAD or PAS? All of these terms have been used by both proponents and opponents.

For this discussion several terms will be used. "Aid in dying" is the term that has emerged as the leading candidate. "Physician assisted death" is also used because it is the assistance of the physician that is currently at issue in the debates. These terms, however, are used to describe the identical conduct. The term "suicide" is not used for reasons specifically addressed below.

Here we focus on aid in dying as allowed in the State of Oregon. There are good reasons for limiting our analysis to that model. Several states have already followed the Oregon design. Current and future debates in the remaining states are likely to be focused on the Oregon Death With Dignity Act. That law was effective in 1997 and has been in use since that time. We have more than a decade and a half of experience with the Oregon law as a reference. Finally, that legislation is a good example of the result requested from those who continue to advocate for aid in dying.

To fully understand and appreciate how aid in dying works in Oregon, obtain a copy of the video "How to Die in Oregon." This 107 minute video is easily available and shows clearly the intent and result of the Oregon law.

We are only discussing cases in which a competent, terminally illl, adult patient requests the physician's assistance in dying. Oregon states it this way:

> "Who may initiate a written request for medication. (1) An adult who is capable, is a resident of Oregon, and has been determined by the attending physician and consult-ing physician to be suffering from a terminal disease, and who has voluntarily expressed his or her wish to die, may make a written request for medication for the purpose of ending his or her life in a humane and dignified man-ner (in accordance with specific procedures and forms)." (Oregon Revised Statutes 127.805 §2.01)

These are the key concepts involved with aid in dying. They involve a competent adult who has been determined to be terminally ill and who has asked the physician to provide the means to end the patient's life quickly and without further suffering. A physician may provide knowledge and prescribe drugs which, when taken by the patient, will cause death. After acquiring the prescription the patient may or may not choose to fill the prescription. If the prescription is filled, the patient may or may not choose to take the drugs.

The Oregon Death With Dignity Act contains many specific "safe-guards" through definitions, requirements, procedures, forms and penalties. A good "plain language" explanation of the Oregon legislation has been promulgated by Compassion and Choices of Oregon and is available on their website.

We are concerned only with those cases which traditionally raise the issue of physician assistance in death. In such cases the patient may say to the physician:

"Doctor, I am dying. You have all tried everything but I am still dying. I do not fear death and I accept the reality of death. I fear this dying process and I wish to have control of my remaining life and death. Please help me to die in a quick and painless way."

One need not discuss these matters with many long practicing physicians before meeting a physician who has encountered such a request. It is only in regard to this patient in this situation that we explore the ultimate question. If you change the facts, then you change the analysis. If you wish to discuss a different patient or different physician action, you change the discussion. And we make this clear because it is the Oregon model of aid in dying we focus upon.

B. Very Few Individuals

It is fair to ask why all of this attention, this feeling, this amount of strident debate is invested in actions that directly affect so few persons. With all that has been said about aid in dying in the past several decades, very few dying individuals reach the point of wanting to hasten their own deaths.

The Oregon Death With Dignity Act requires reports and the State maintains statistics. The annual report for 2013 shows that since the law became effective in 1997, a total of 1,173 people have had prescriptions written and 752 patients have died in accordance with the statute. Compare that number with the nearly 500,000 persons who have died in Oregon since 1998.

These numbers are not surprising. Most human beings will never seek to hasten their own deaths. Nearly all human beings fight for life and resist death with all their might. We know this.

In Oregon and elsewhere one can read obituaries and find a daily reference to an individual who has died "after a courageous battle with cancer." But a few of us do request aid in dying and the issue has been argued passionately throughout the world for quite some time. There are several reasons for this.

First, we are considering life and death, literally. Thinking about death requires us to confront fears. Stare at the word for a moment.

DEATH

Simply confronting this word causes a reaction in most persons. Fear or dread is the feeling. Because it involves death the subject generates intense feelings and challenges fundamental beliefs. When fundamental beliefs and strong feelings conflict, heated debate usually follows.

Second, there is death and then there is dying. Many envision (or hope for) their death as slipping away peacefully in the night or fading to black with family and friends at the bedside. But the reality is often quite different. Medical knowledge and modern technology allow us to postpone death. We have read and heard stories of a long, drawn-out dying process. We may have seen a loved one or friend suffer terribly while dying. Regardless of how few might choose to hasten their own deaths, however, most of us are quite concerned about how our dying might occur.

Third, these patients have specifically told us they choose death to continued life. The fact that some individuals express this unusual desire causes us to wonder why and whether it is right or wrong. We cannot avoid this difficult subject.

C. Is Aid In Dying "Suicide?"

Should we say that terminally ill patients who request and receive assistance from their doctor and hasten their own deaths have committed "suicide?" Is the term "suicide" appropriate? Does the term help or hinder our quest for a clear and thoughtful answer?

One effect of using the term "suicide" is to immediately include these patients within a category of deaths that most of us consider tragic. What are your feelings and thoughts when you hear that a person has committed suicide?

You can use terms as weapons and you can use the term "suicide" as a weapon in the discussion of aid in dying. Words mean something, of course. Beyond meaning, words can generate feelings, even strong feelings. Feelings shape thoughts and conclusions regarding aid in dying. The use of the term "suicide" can prejudice the discussion from the beginning and confuse rather than clarify the debate. "You mean you support suicide?" "We simply cannot have a doctor participating in the suicide of her patient!" Each statement has a negative connotation and those statements are used to express strong disapproval. However, one may very well oppose assisting "suicide" and still support the legality of "aid in dying."

There are several significant arguments against using the term "suicide." The first and most sensible is to simply recognize that we often use different terms to describe different circumstances. For example: A shoots and kills B. What term should we use to describe this act of killing? It may be first degree murder, second degree murder, voluntary manslaughter, involuntary manslaughter, justifiable homicide or self defense. Which is it? In all six the basic facts are the same: A shoots and kills B.

To determine what term to use we examine the circumstances? Who were they? What were they doing? What were they thinking? And so on. Because we recognize the different circumstances and intent we use different terms to describe the act. It makes sense to recognize those differences. It makes sense to recognize the different circumstances and intent surrounding aid in dying.

Consider six further cases in which individuals choose a course of action resulting in their death.

A Jehovah's Witness needs a life saving blood transfusion. She understands her critical medical situation and that the consequence of her refusal will be death. Because of her strongly held religious beliefs, however, she refuses the transfusion and dies.

A patient has been undergoing life saving dialysis. At this point, and all things considered, he decides to quit his dialysis. He knows that without continued dialysis he will die. He dies.

A Marine and his squad are in a defensive position and under attack. An enemy grenade lands in their midst. He knows well what a grenade can do. Knowing this he throws his body over the grenade. He dies.

A chronically depressed but physically healthy 30-year old despondent over his personal relationships and financial difficulties sees no escape from his problems and shoots himself. He dies.

A Buddhist monk opposes the war raging in his country. As a political protest he sits and refuses to eat. He dies.

A competent, dying patient is suffering and seeks to avoid the continuing and prolonged dying process. She requests the assistance of her physician. Her physician prescribes drugs. She eventually chooses to consume them. She dies.

In each of these cases the individual had a choice between continued life and death. In each case the person acted to bring about his or her premature death. Are they all "suicides?" Some? Which and why?

Theologians and philosophers spend hours discussing these issues. They will start pointing out the differences in these cases. They will argue differences in action and intent. Was it "active" or "passive?" Did someone "do something" or simply "let it happen?" Was the intent to die or something else? But, fundamentally, in each case the individual had options and chose a course of action they knew would bring about their death. While most would have no difficulty referring to the 30 year old as a "suicide," do we want to label the other five deaths "suicides?" Should all of the death certificates declare that the person died as a "suicide?"

There are other reasons to question the use of the term "suicide."

Many have referred to the suicides we wish to prevent as "irrational self-destruction." This seems sensible. But are all dying individuals who seek aid in dying involved in "irrational self-destruction?" Are the Jehovah's Witness and the Marine involved in "irrational self destruction?" We allow that religious choice and we present posthumous medals for such heroism. Again, who were they? What were their situations? Why did they act? And so on.

Consider the Buddhist monk. Wouldn't this be considered a "political suicide?" Yet it is ethically and legally proper for a dying patient to voluntarily refuse further food and liquids in the quest to hasten the dying process. We do not refer to those cases as "suicides." How tricky our language can be.

Many have pointed out another significant difference. With aid in dying we have a person who wants to live but who is dying. With suicide we have a person who could live but wants to die.

We might ask the families of those who have requested aid in dying if they think their loved one "committed suicide." Is this how they perceive the death of their family member? Are they likely to believe that their father "died of pancreatic cancer" or "committed suicide?"

There are many individuals and organizations dedicated to preventing suicides. If aid in dying is "suicide," shouldn't those organizations have an interest in preventing these deaths? A search of their literature and purposes can find no references to aid in dying or any desire to become involved with aid in dying cases because they are suicides to be prevented.

Finally, there is a popular expression that refers to suicides. "Suicide is a permanent solution to a temporary problem." Does this apply to the terminally ill patient who requests aid in dying? It is true that the dying process is temporary. It will end. What is the proper solution to the temporary problem of dying?

Some opponents of aid in dying accuse those who avoid using the term "suicide" of "avoiding the facts." For example, the United States Conference of Catholic Bishops declares:

> "Proponents . . . avoid terms such as 'assisting suicide' and instead use euphemisms such as 'aid in dying.' (P)lain speaking is needed to strip away this veneer and uncover what is at stake, for this agenda promotes neither free choice nor compassion."

Is it "plain speaking" to declare that the 30-year old, the dialysis patient, and the dying patient requesting aid in dying are all simply "suicides?" We could declare them all to be "suicides." But, just as with our shooting example, we see the clear differences and that those situations are better communicated with different terms.

Words can mean anything we want them to mean. You can decide if the term "suicide" is appropriate for these cases or whether sufficient differences exist to distinguish the circumstances, action, intent, and the terms used to describe them. It is a matter of linguistic choice. But the choice should make sense and help in the communication of ideas. The choice here is not to discuss "suicides." Here we discuss individuals who are dying, rational, and who seek assistance in hastening their impending deaths. It is about timing.

You will encounter individuals and groups who insist on using the term "suicide." Generally, those who continue to use the term "suicide" do so because it is an effective weapon in the battle to oppose aid in dying. Regardless of terms, however, the arguments remain the same. And there are no arguments sufficient to justify the criminalization of aid in dying in American society.

D. Current Legal Status in the United States

We will not take time to present a history of aid in dying. Many others have done so and there are numerous sources one can consult to learn the long history of efforts to legalize aid in dying in the United States. Here we limit our remarks to note that aid in dying is specifically permitted in only five states. By vote in Oregon, Washington and Vermont and by action of the courts in Montana and New Mexico. (At the time of this writing the New Mexico case was on appeal.)

In the United States the legal status of aid in dying is considered a State issue and is controlled by state law. This is why the issue is being raised separately in state after state. (You may check the website of Compassion and Choices for information regarding your state.)

At this time no state makes it a crime to commit suicide. This is true whether the person uses deadly gas, a shotgun, drives off a cliff, or involves the assistance of a physician. The individual has not committed the crime of "suicide." It is assisting a suicide that remains criminal. Aiding or abetting or encouraging a suicide is a crime in many states. For example, California Penal Code Section 401 provides: "Every person who deliberately aids, or advises, or encourages another to commit suicide, is guilty of a felony."

This is understandable. Most of us consider suicides to be tragedies. They seem to be the result of unfortunate circumstances. The suicidal person does not appear competent to make a rational life and death decision. Because it is "irrational self-destruction," it should be prevented. And because we seek to prevent suicides we seek to prevent others from aiding or encouraging suicides. This is also true in Oregon.

In most states physicians who provide knowledge and prescriptions for lethal drugs, even at the request of competent, dying patients risk prosecutions under those laws prohibiting aiding suicides.

E. The Legislative Solution

What is the way out? How do Oregon and other states distinguish aid in dying from the cases of irrational self-destruction we still seek to prevent? This distinction is really quite easy.

The Oregon statute simply declares that actions taken in accordance with the Death With Dignity Act "shall not, for any purpose, constitute suicide, assisted suicide, mercy killing or homicide, under the law." The people of Oregon see sufficient differences in circumstances and intent to exclude aid in dying from the category of "suicides." If physicians act in accordance with the procedures and safeguards of the Act, they may work with all patients in managing dying and death. The crime of aiding and abetting a suicide has not been committed.

Whether aid in dying should be permitted or prohibited is a public policy issue. It is not a medical decision to be made by physicians. It is not a legal decision to be made by lawyers. It is not a religious or ethical decision to be made by theologians and bioethicists.

Aid in dying is a social policy issue to be made by all of us. It is to be made by you and the rest of our voting population. Since we all have a say in public policy, this discussion is for everyone. It is for both supporters and opponents. It is for everyone who is thoughtful and seeking in good faith to understand the issues and reach an honest conclusion.

F.   The Ultimate Question

The ultimate question and the only issue of concern here is: Should a competent, dying adult be permitted to receive the assistance of a physician to hasten death? The question involves criminality.

This ultimate question can be presented in multiple ways. For example, should aid in dying as permitted in Oregon be permitted in your state?

We can also highlight the issue with two very different statements. An opponent of aid in dying might declare: "I think aid in dying is wrong and I will never choose such a death." She would also argue: "I think aid in dying is wrong and no one should ever be allowed to choose such a death." Our concern is the difference between the personal point of view expressed in the first statement and the desire for criminal penalties expressed in the second. The first is acceptable. The second is unacceptable.

G.   There Are Only Three Categories of Objections

Every argument against aid in dying falls within one of the following three categories.

1) It is wrong for a dying individual to hasten death.
2) Even if it is not wrong to hasten death, it is wrong for a physician to assist.
3) Even if it is not wrong to hasten death with the help of a physician, aid in dying will cause more harm than good.

Another way of stating the three categories of opposition is that aid in dying should be prohibited because:

1) It is morally wrong.
2) It is contrary to the professional ethics of physicians.
3) It will cause more harm than good.

We will investigate each of these three categories in turn.

H.   Is Death the Worst Thing That Can Happen To Us?

Here is a final introductory question. Is death the worst thing that can happen to a human being? It often appears that many who oppose aid in dying believe this to be true.

We know, as individuals and as a society, this is not always true. Death can be a friend - a welcomed event. We are familiar with these deaths. We describe them as "the best thing" or "wonderfully quick." Seeing a loved one or a friend or even a stranger experience a long and painful dying, perhaps aided and abetted by medicine and machines, is itself an excruciating experience.

It is also clear that as a society we do not consider individual human life to be our highest value. We can think of numerous instances in which we value other things more than continued human lives. From war to speed limits we make societal choices we know will lead to avoidable human deaths. We do so because we think the values behind those choices rank higher than some individual human lives. Yet we see arguments opposing aid in dying that only appear explainable if death is the worst thing that can happen to a dying human being.

We will ask this question at various points in analyzing the opposition to aid in dying.

Part Two

Is It Wrong to Hasten Death?

Is it right or wrong for a dying individual to hasten death?

It is important to consider this fundamental question because many argue that intentionally hastening death is morally wrong and, because that is true, aid in dying should be prohibited. If it can be shown that it is wrong, perhaps we can properly prohibit such action.

Why do some argue it is wrong for a dying individual to hasten death?

First, we must understand how human beings generally reach conclusions regarding what is right and wrong. Most of us have never taken a course in ethics but all of us have opinions regarding what is right and wrong. Second, we must understand the nature of ethical inquiry and whether ethics can resolve our question.

We will explore both of these areas to demonstrate that one cannot criminalize aid in dying because it is morally wrong or ethically incorrect.

A. Feelings and Beliefs

When we have conflicting views of right and wrong, how do we generally resolve our differences? Is it by reference to ethical theory? When there is conflict, is it because different persons are applying different ethical principles, one of which is correct and one of which is incorrect? When we seek to change another person's opinion relating to whether or not a particular act is right/ethical or wrong/unethical, do we attempt to persuade them to adopt a different philosophy?

Most often when we want to change another's conclusions we spend time trying to change (1) their feelings toward the action, (2) their beliefs which relate to the conduct, or (3) their assessment of the consequences of the action.

Both feelings and religious beliefs are center stage in the debates concerning aid in dying. Many never get beyond them. And while they are quite often the primary reason for an individual's conclusions, they are the worst reasons for deciding public policy. And it is easy to understand why they are a bad foundation for public policy. The following comments relating to emotions and religious beliefs should be obvious to most but they must be continually emphasized. It is difficult to underestimate the influence our feelings and beliefs have upon our judgments of what is right or wrong.

Feelings - Generally, if conduct makes one feel good, joyous, compassionate (any "positive" emotional response), the action is thought to be "right." On the other hand, if the action makes us feel sad, angry or disgusted (any "negative" emotional response), then the action is considered to be "wrong."

When we have an emotional reaction to actions we often challenge others based upon those reactions. For example:

- "I am horrified by what he did and it shouldn't be allowed."
- "How can you think that is right? You ought to be outraged at the lack of care."
- "That is awful. Don't you have compassion for those people?"
- "I'm ashamed of myself. That was wrong."

We have feelings and we challenge others based upon those feelings. But when we say these things we are doing nothing more than asserting the other person is not feeling what we feel and he or she should be experiencing the same emotions as we are. And, of course, if they did feel the way we feel, their conclusion would be different. It would be like ours. But what if they simply do not feel the way we do? "You say I should be sad about this, but I'm not." "I'd like to feel good about this situation, but I don't." Where does the debate go from there?

One would think it would be quite simple for individuals to understand that their personal feelings regarding conduct are not sufficient reason to criminalize the conduct. But it is not simple as is demonstrated in nearly all public debates concerning social issues. While most of us do understand and appreciate this point, it must constantly be emphasized and made clear. An individual's feelings or a majority's feelings alone cannot establish what is right or wrong and cannot properly justify criminalizing conduct for everyone.

Religious Beliefs - A second primary source for judgments of right and wrong are our irrational beliefs. Here we focus on beliefs which result in appeals to religious authority. As with arguments based upon emotions, appeals to authority remove the subject from the realms of rational thought and discourse. They also bring to mind the well known bumper sticker: "God said it. I believe it. That settles it."

We often hear arguments which appeal to religious authority.

- "You are incorrect. The Bible does prohibit blood transfusions."
- "Gay marriage is wrong because Billy Graham says the Bible says it is wrong."
- "Those who support aid in dying are wrong because the Koran prohibits suicide."

When we make these appeals to authority we are doing nothing more than asserting the other person does not believe what we believe and they should believe the same as we do. If they did share our beliefs then they would have the same attitude toward the conduct as we do. But what if they simply do not believe the way we do? "You say I should believe the Bible is God's word but I just don't believe that." "You argue that all Buddhists must be vegetarians to be true Buddhists but I don't believe that is true." "The Pope may say that is wrong but my Rabbi says otherwise." From this impasse, where do we take the discussion?

If you are a Christian do you want to spend time arguing with a Hindu that you should be bound by the authority of his holy books? For you, they are irrelevant. Consider that even if everyone were Christian and believed that the Bible stood for the word of God there are still problems. Although there are some who think otherwise, there can be no literal meaning of the Bible. It must be interpreted by someone. Do you want to be bound by someone else's interpretation which is different from yours?

If you still believe that your religious beliefs are sufficient to establish that aid in dying is wrong and should be criminal, consider the following situation. Here is an example that should make this point obvious to everyone. Suppose Jehovah's Witnesses gain a majority in your State. They may be very pleasant neighbors but do you think they could properly criminalize blood transfusions? They would do so, of course, because blood transfusions are forbidden by God's word as contained in the Bible.

If you do not believe the majority could properly do this, then you understand the obvious problems with criminalizing aid in dying based upon religious authority. Although often heard in our neighborhoods, religious authority arguments are absolutely irrelevant when considering what public policy should be in our secular society. These arguments in the debate over public policy are, quite frankly, un-American.

Some actions are condemned on both fronts. They are declared "wrong" both because of strong emotional reactions to the conduct and because they conflict with religious beliefs. Gays and lesbians have heard it often. "Your actions are against the word of God and disgusting and wrong!"

You are familiar with emotional and religious arguments and they can be heard in any conversation involving important social issues. They occur because this is how we naturally think. We naturally link feelings and beliefs with labels of right and wrong.

For human beings feelings and beliefs are fundamental to what we are. A feeling may be considered inappropriate or difficult to understand, but it exists and it leads us to certain conclusions. A religious belief may be unorthodox, but it exists and it influences our conclusions.

It does no good to deny the existence, validity, or effect of feelings and beliefs. It is most valuable to recognize their existence and what naturally flows from them. And while feelings and beliefs are both irrational, "irrational" does not equate with "bad" or "stupid." Feelings and beliefs are irrational because what we feel and what we believe are not things we rationally reflect upon and exert our will to make a considered choice.

B.   A Secular, Pluralistic Society

Because we often have feelings and beliefs that are quite different a further reminder always seems to be necessary when we discuss highly charged social issues. It is as though many of us have forgotten our elementary school history lessons. We live in a secular, pluralistic society. What does this mean?

We are a pluralistic society. We feel differently. We believe differently. We act differently. Many times we feel, believe and act very differently.

We are a secular society. We do not have defined religious beliefs imposed upon us. Our foundational document speaks to this when declaring we will enjoy free exercise of religion. We should not fear jail because our beliefs conflict with those in power. Or those of the majority. We know that even in the 21st century there are other societies who think differently. In some areas of the world if you do not profess orthodox beliefs you may be jailed or even killed.

We were intended to be a secular, pluralistic society. This entire discussion assumes we want to live in such a society. It assumes we want to live in the United States, under our Constitution, and in peace with our very diverse neighbors.

It is sometimes difficult to tolerate others acting foolishly and irresponsibly. One thing is certain. We cannot live together in peace and enjoy the freedom to pursue our own happiness unless we have a high level of tolerance for others and they for us.

For all of these reasons we must eliminate all arguments based upon personal feelings or religious beliefs from the debates. In our diverse society, neither can properly establish that aid in dying is wrong and should be prohibited. We must attempt some other means to reach a proper answer to our ultimate question regarding aid in dying.

The next sensible step is to attempt to answer our question through ethical inquiry. Can ethical inquiry establish whether it is right or wrong for a dying individual to hasten death?

C.   Can Ethical Inquiry Resolve the Issue?

Ethics is the discipline of philosophy that deals with what is right and what is wrong. In "doing ethics" we attempt by critical thought, or disciplined puzzling, or rational discourse, to resolve controversies concerning what constitutes right action. "Bioethics" is simply the process of ethics applied to issues involved with the delivery of health care and the biomedical disciplines. The issue of aid in dying falls within the realm of bioethics.

Engaging in ethical inquiry is seeking dialogue with others who are sincere and acting in good faith. We are searching together for the best reasons for a position or a conclusion. We attempt to define and clarify the issues. We ask what do you mean by that? Is a position consistent? If an argument cannot be applied consistently it may not be the best argument. Is it logical? Does the conclusion properly follow from the premises? Is it based in reality or does it seem fanciful and groundless? Does an argument show good sense and sound judgment? Is it sensible? Sensible is an excellent word. We will use if often. All of these concepts apply when one is attempting in good faith to puzzle through a difficult ethical issue such as aid in dying.

There are two important reasons for doing ethics when considering issues such as aid in dying. Keep both in mind.

1)   We simply must go beyond personal feelings and beliefs in our public ethics.

We make judgments relating to what is right and wrong for at least two important purposes. First, we make judgments to guide our own conduct. Judgments for this purpose can be labeled our "personal ethics." Second, as members of a community we participate in making judgments which will bind us all. These determinations can be labeled our "public ethics." In a very real sense our criminal laws constitute our public ethics. They set out what conduct we will and will not allow.

Judgments based upon personal feelings or beliefs may be sufficient to guide our own conduct but there are obvious reasons why we cannot rely upon either to govern everyone's conduct.

2) We must seek an alternative to the use of force.

We "do ethics" as an alternative to the use of force. Most of us do not generally consider "the law" as using force against our neighbors. But criminal laws authorize arrest and jailing. If it is illegal we allow the use of power and force against individuals who act contrary to what the law requires.

If I think something is wrong and no one should be allowed to do that thing, and the use of force against others does not trouble me (and I have the power), then I do not need to consider your feelings or your beliefs or to do ethics. I do not need to reason with you. I can simply use force to enforce my view of things. But if I am troubled by the use of force against others (and by others against me), then I will seek to resolve differences by nonviolent means.

Ethical inquiry is of interest only to those who are troubled by the use of force against others and the possible use of force by others against them. These considerations apply not simply to individuals but to large democratic majorities. At this time in most of the United States our public policy is to use force against those who participate in aid in dying. We authorize the use of force regardless of their feelings, beliefs or ethical conclusions.

D. Ethical Theories, Principles and Values

The attempt here is to be concise, sensible and understandable so that this handbook is useful for those involved in the debate. The intent is not to produce a history or survey of ethics or volumes of difficult ethical concepts.

It is necessary, however, to say something about the nature of ethics because we ask whether ethical inquiry can properly resolve our questions regarding hastening death. Further, and importantly, ethical inquiry is a part of the debate as some "ethical experts" use their expertise to declare that aid in dying is wrong and should remain criminal. They still exert influence when the matter is put to public vote.

We will keep this short and simple for three important reasons. First, this is all we need to know about ethical inquiry to understand its application to the dilemma of aid in dying. Second, if we set out the very best ethical analysis that can be conceived it will not resolve this dilemma. Third, a large portion of the ethical analysis of aid in dying fundamentally fails to appreciate what aid in dying is really about.

Ethical Theories

When we do ethics we organize our thoughts and propose different ideas with the hope that they will lead us to a proper conclusion. We use tools. We can use the ethical tools of theories, principles and values to help resolve ethical dilemmas.

Ethical theories are broad statements of how to determine what is right or wrong. We cannot attempt even a cursory review of the numerous ethical theories that have been proposed over the centuries. This is not a scholarly philosophy textbook in which we study and compare the views of Plato with those of Kant with those of Hobbes or Mill or make any attempt to judge which ethical theory is superior. In the simplest way here are the two main general theories which demonstrate that no single ethical theory can resolve the many conflicts that arise in human society and modern bioethics (including aid in dying).

There are utilitarian theories which tell us that one ought conduct one-self so as to bring about a greater amount of good than evil. We should act so that the consequences of the action are more good than bad. This sounds sensible. These are known as teleological or "consequentialist" theories. We devote a fair amount of time to "consequence" arguments directed against aid in dying in Part 4. They are a substantial part of the aid in dying debate.

There are deontological or duty based theories. These concepts are generally traced to Immanuel Kant (1724-1804). Duty based theories maintain that we have certain moral duties *regardless of the consequences*. Kant declared one should always act in such a way that your rule of conduct should become a universal law. For Kant, we have strict duties and things we must and must not do. For example, we should treat all persons as an end and never merely as a means. We should not lie and we should never kill an innocent person regardless of the circumstances. That is your duty. That is what is right irrespective of the consequences.

There are many variations and subtleties to both of these schools of thought and there are other schools advancing other ethical theories. A full study of ethics is a daunting task. Why are there so many different ethical theories? Are we searching for the ethical holy grail? Are human beings seeking a unified theory of ethics - *the* theory which we can always apply to give us the right answer? But there is no such theory.

No ethical theory will allow us to resolve all questions of right and wrong. But different theories are useful in different situations.

We might want to apply utilitarian concepts to help design the "right" way to share limited resources - a public health program, for example. We might proceed on the theory that our limited resources should provide "the greatest amount of good for the greatest number." That is the consequence we desire. That sounds sensible.

Perhaps we can agree that using that particular ethical theory is the right way to proceed. Then again, you might argue we have a duty to provide more resources to particular classes of persons - mothers and young children, perhaps - with the consequence that a higher number of elderly would go without.

At the same time we may not want to stand by "the greatest good for the greatest number" when considering another area of bioethical concern - the proper way to harvest and distribute organs for transplantation.

To achieve the greatest good for the greatest number we might kill a healthy person so five others could live. After all, what's the loss of one life compared to saving the lives of five others? Do the math. No, in that case we would declare ourselves "deontologists" and assert that we have a duty to never use an innocent person for the benefit of another regardless of the consequences. (But what about a properly convicted murderer?)

How does this apply to aid in dying? In regard to consequences, if we all agreed that permitting aid in dying has terrible consequences and produces more harm than good, we could properly conclude that aid in dying should be prohibited. But we do not all agree and this cannot be shown. Many of us believe it produces good and no harm.

In regard to duties, if we all agreed that every one has a duty not to hasten death, then we could properly conclude it is wrong to hasten death regardless of the consequences. And we could properly conclude that it is wrong to assist such a death. But we do not all agree. Some of us believe our duty is to relieve human suffering or to allow freedom of human choice and that aid in dying is consistent with that duty.

Different ethical theories can help us resolve different ethical dilemmas. They can give us rational reasons and sensible justification for a conclusion. However, no ethical theory can resolve (1) all dilemmas or (2) any particular ethical dilemma unless we agree on the applicability of the theory to the situation.

Ethical Principles

Beyond ethical theories, ethical principles also exist. We can consider ethical principles in our search for answers. These are concepts we can keep in mind as we attempt to determine what is right and wrong.

An early and very well known book in bioethics entitled *Principles of Biomedical Ethics* (Tom L. Beauchamp and James F. Childress) sets out four major principles to guide us in resolving bioethical problems. It is thought if one keeps these principles in mind, it will guide the journey to what is right in medicine. Again, we do not go far down this road. We go only far enough to see the conclusion. The four principles are:

Autonomy - "Autonomy" from the Greek means "self rule." We generally understand what is meant by this term. Much theology, philosophy and legal theory has been based upon the idea that an individual should have the ability to control his own life. This sounds sensible. But, then again, what do we do with the concept of autonomy when we lie to a patient with the use of placebos or involuntarily treat others?

Nonmaleficence - We should never intentionally harm another. This sounds sensible. But, then again, what do we mean by "harm" and what if we disagree concerning what amounts to harm?

Beneficence - Not only should we not harm others, we should take action which is beneficial to others. We should attempt to do good for others. This sounds sensible. Then again, who should decide what is beneficial to others?

Justice - We should attempt to "be just" and to "do justice." We think of fairness, equality and lawfulness. This sounds sensible. But can you define "justice?"

Do you agree or disagree with these well recognized "principles of bioethics?" Let individuals control their own actions unless it produces some real harm to others. Do no harm. Do good. Be just.

Who does not agree with these principles? The atheist, the Rabbi and the Muslim all have very different world views but they all can heartedly agree with these concepts. But do they resolve all conflicts? They do not.

One can consider these ethical principles when confronted with a problem. We can ask which principle or principles apply? Do they help guide us to an answer? Do they state a reason for choosing X over Y? "This rule allows for personal freedom and it is right." "That causes harm and it is wrong." "That is not fair for all and is incorrect."

Unfortunately, however, principles often conflict. For example, the principle of autonomy is overridden by the principle of beneficence when involuntarily confining a mentally ill individual who is considered dangerous to himself or others. Would we be doing good or causing harm if we permitted payment to organ donors? Does aid in dying cause harm or is it beneficial? Does the second or third principle apply? Or does the first principle trump all?

As with ethical theories, ethical principles can also give us rational reasons to justify our conclusions and different principles can help us resolve different ethical dilemmas. No ethical principle, however, can resolve (1) all dilemmas or (2) any particular dilemma unless we agree on the applicability of the principle to the situation.

Values

We all have values, things we think are valuable. Traditional values include truth, beauty, wisdom, fairness and freedom. There are many other values - peace, love, courage, curiosity, patience, compassion, forgiveness, tolerance, wisdom, intelligence, honesty, humor, harmony, tenderness, love, life, health, passion, pleasure, and on and on. Again, the Buddhist and the Christian may have different world views but may very well share the same values.

Our values come from varied sources and we will not here attempt a discussion of the source of our values. It can be parents, teachers, priests, tribe, or experience. As with our irrational feelings and beliefs, it is not important to know where they come from, only to recognize that they exist and they lead us to certain conclusions.

We apply these values when we attempt to make determinations of what is right and wrong. But the problem in applying our values is the same as with feelings and beliefs. We often have different values. And even if we share the same values, we may rank them differently. "I think personal freedom is what we should value here but you insist that it is duty to others." "You think equality is the highest value but I think recognizing merit is of higher value in this situation." Where do we go from there?

We do ethics. We apply different concepts to help us sort out right from wrong. We consider theories, principles and values. Each and all can give us reason to justify our conclusions in a particular situation. But none of them can do so all of the time. How do we determine which theory or principle or value trumps in any given case? We think about where such and such a theory leads and ask if it is appropriate. Is it sensible? We explore several principles and do the same thing. Does this principle fit here and does it make sense? We go back to values and see if they apply to the situation. How many values are involved in this situation? Do they conflict? How do they conflict? Is one of higher value than the others?

We can do this together. Maybe, just maybe, we will discuss the applicability of various theories, principles and values and agree. We will all come to the same conclusion that theory A and principle B apply and, therefor, X is right and Y is wrong. But what if we do not agree? You insist on one theory and I argue another. You say we always have a duty to do X but I don't think so. You say the principle of autonomy is directly applicable here but I think justice overrides it in this case. You say the highest value is individual freedom but I don't think so.

In regard to ethical inquiry and aid in dying, no ethical theory, principle or statement of value can establish that it is wrong for a dying individual to hasten their own death unless we agree upon the application of the theory, principle or value. And we do not agree.

Examine any ethical analysis of aid in dying and seek out where the author's feelings and beliefs are seeping (if not flooding) through. What theory do they promote and why? What principle do they rely upon and why? What are their values? Are these the only theories, principles and values worth considering and do they conclusively trump all others? Of course they do not.

You may agree with someone's reasoning and conclusions that aid in dying is wrong. That agreement would be sufficient in itself to justify your conclusion that it would be wrong for you to hasten your own death. It could also give you reason to think that it is wrong for others to hasten their own deaths. But it utterly fails to establish that aid in dying is wrong and should be prohibited for everyone.

We can argue forever. Some of us might change sides. We might be convinced one theory or principle or value is more important than others. We might even go back and forth in our conclusions. But what if after hours, days, months, years and centuries of ethical inquiry and dialogue we still do not agree whether it is right or wrong for a dying individual to hasten his own death? Of course, this is exactly where we are today. We have reached the limits of ethical inquiry.

E. The Limits of Ethical Inquiry

We do ethics because it is our nature to puzzle things out. Ethical inquiry can help us organize our thoughts and give us sensible reasons and justification for conduct. Ethical discussions can help us think through areas of disagreement. But there are very real limits upon rational thought to determine what is right. If ethical inquiry could resolve issues involving feelings, beliefs and values, then we would no longer be arguing whether paying organ donors, gay marriage, abortion, embryonic research or aid in dying is right or wrong.

While we often follow Aristotle's lead and classify ourselves as "rational animals," all adults should know we are only partially rational. Yes, we have the capacity to be rational and we do act rationally. But we are also very much irrational. We know we make judgments based upon irrational feelings and beliefs.

We try to establish with certainty what is right and what is wrong through ethical inquiry but it often leaves us lost and confused. If ethics cannot lead us to the right answer regarding what is right and wrong, what is ethics?

Ethics (bioethics) is the attempt by semi-rational beings to rationalize that which is essentially irrational.

This definition is not offered in jest. It is intended to again emphasize the effect our irrational beliefs and emotions have upon our judgments regarding what is right and what is wrong.

Something causes one person joy and another sorrow. Why? One believes God forbids action and one does not. Why? Some people apply different theories, principles and values in determining whether conduct is right or wrong. Why? Some think it is consequences that matter while others believe we have certain duties regardless of the consequences. Who is correct? Some think the principle of autonomy applies and others declare that the principle of beneficence controls. Who is right? One thinks life is the highest value while others declare freedom of choice the ultimate value. Which is "righter?" We and our neighbors disagree. Why?

The fundamental effect of our irrational feelings and beliefs upon our judgments may be the single most important thing to remember when attempting to comprehend the nature of ethical dilemmas and the endless and often heated debates in the search for what is "right" public policy. For even as we attempt to have rational discussions our irrational feelings and beliefs are active participants in forming our ultimate conclusions concerning what theory or principle or values apply. (The foremost example in American society is, of course, the debate surrounding abortion.)

In attempting to establish what is "right" on any particular issue we must be prepared to confront the ways in which human beings actually consider matters of right and wrong. We must be prepared to confront deeply felt irrational emotions, strongly held irrational beliefs and the different application of theories and values which are influenced by those irrational emotions and beliefs.

We must understand and appreciate that no one can establish with certainty what is ultimately true. There is no one who has lived or living today who can tell us with absolute certainty why there are one hundred billion galaxies or the meaning of human existence. There are no experts who can do this and we will never agree that there is an expert who can perform this task. If there were, we could simply look to that individual to tell us what values are higher than other values and what constitutes the good. Because we do not have such an ultimate authority, we must learn to accept diversity and uncertainty if we wish to live in peace with one another.

F. Diversity, Uncertainty, Freedom, Peace, Toleration

We are diverse. We see the diversity in our neighborhood. We are often uncertain whether something is right or wrong. We want to be free to make our own choices. So do our neighbors. If we want to live in peace with our neighbors we all must be able to accept both our diversity and our uncertainty. If we want to refrain from using force we must have a good deal of toleration for the feelings, beliefs and actions of others. But let us be clear. We are not required to tolerate others. If we are not troubled by the use of force and we have the power, we can simply make conduct illegal and use force against those who disagree. Of course, we must also by prepared for others to use force against us if their feelings, beliefs or values are different from ours.

The "morality of mutual respect" is a phrase from *The Foundations of Bioethics* by H. T. Englehardt, Jr. For Englehardt tolerating the moral views of others is itself a moral issue. Englehardt rightly points out that in a free society individuals will reach different conclusions regarding what is good and bad and what is right and wrong. This is obvious to us. And individuals will choose different courses of action based upon their differing decisions regarding what is right or wrong. This is also obvious. Further, some of those decisions we will consider tragic. We wonder how could anyone think that is right. "With all that has been said about the dangers of smoking during the past forty years, how can anyone still smoke a pack a day? That is so wrong." We would never make that terrible decision.

We can state a dozen or a hundred things other people choose to do even though we think their decisions are terrible decisions. (And they could, no doubt, point out a few things we do that they believe are misguided and wrong.) But living in a neighborhood, a city and a state where others make different and sometimes tragic choices is the price we must pay if we wish to live in a free and peaceful society. Englehardt states it this way:

> "The purchase price of freedom is tragedy and diversity. It is tragedy because individuals in their freedom will choose in ways that others find to be ill considered and harmful. Such choices will lead to an untidy diversity of competing moral viewpoints, often making common actions in many areas impossible. Because one is obliged to tolerate such tragedy and diversity, the moral life becomes an ambiguous undertaking. One must often tolerate on moral grounds that which one must condemn on moral grounds."

We are diverse. We are uncertain regarding ultimate truth. We wish to live in peace and be free to make our own decisions. We must also tolerate the choices of others even though we believe those choices to be tragic.

No one can establish through ethical inquiry that it is wrong for a dying individual to hasten death. And there is no justification for the criminalization of aid in dying because that end of life choice is "wrong."

Finally, in the consideration of ethics we might also quickly mention one last ethical concept. "Do unto others as you would have them do unto you." This simple statement encapsulates much of what has just been stated.

We next consider the role of the physician.

Part Three

Is It Wrong for a Physician to Assist?

What about the role of the physician? Even if it is not wrong for a dying patient to hasten death, is it wrong for a physician to assist as allowed in Oregon?

This discussion is primarily for those physicians and others who agree with the position of the American Medical Association (AMA) that aid in dying is contrary to medical ethics.

Even in 2014 and more than sixteen years experience in Oregon the AMA continues to repeat its 1994 position. AMA Opinion 2.211 regarding "Physician-Assisted Suicide" states in part:

> "It is understandable, though tragic, that some patients in extreme duress - such as those suffering from a terminal, painful, debilitating illness - may come to decide that death is preferable to life. However, allowing physicians to partici-pate in assisted suicide would cause more harm than good. Physician-assisted suicide is fundamentally incompat-ible with the physician's role as healer, would be difficult or impossible to control, and would pose serious societal risks."

It is somewhat understandable why the AMA adopted that position twenty years ago. There was much fear and speculation at that time. It is difficult to understand how that statement stands unchanged in 2014.

Is it the position of the AMA that in Oregon and Washington aid in dying has been difficult or impossible to control? Has it posed serious societal risks to the citizens of the northwest? Has aid in dying caused more harm than good? If there is evidence that these things are true, what is the evidence? If there is not evidence, then the AMA cannot in good faith continue to maintain such statements.

It must be noted that other medical associations support this end of life choice. Those organizations include the American Medical Women's Association, the American Medical Students Association, the American College of Legal Medicine and the American Public Health Association.

In any event, does the opposition of some doctors justify the criminalization of aid in dying? It does not and it cannot. This public policy is not a medical decision.

Here we discuss the historic moral distinctions relied upon in medicine to oppose assisted death and show that they have no application to aid in dying. We also ask the important and most relevant question: Is aid in dying "fundamentally incompatible with the physician's role?"

A. Historic Moral Distinctions Do Not Apply

Discussions of medical ethics and death nearly always involve two historic moral distinctions. The first is the distinction between active and passive - the physician doing something or doing nothing. The second distinction involves the intent of the physician - intent to relieve suffering or cause death. A good amount of the bioethical literature relating to aid in dying and the role of the physician concerns whether these distinctions are important or not. Here we simply point out that these historic debates do not apply to aid in dying as permitted in the Oregon model.

1. Acting to Cause Death or Allowing to Die?

The first historic distinction concerns whether the physician is active or passive. The doctor may do nothing and simply allow the patient to die from the underlying medical causes. Or, the doctor may do something which causes the patient to die. It is argued by some that there is a significant moral difference between acts which permit death and acts which cause death.

It is this distinction theologians and the AMA rely upon to allow physicians to withdraw life saving treatment from patients knowing this will bring death but at the same time prohibit physicians from taking any action to cause the patient's death.

Is there a moral distinction between the two? Arguments go both ways. Some argue there is no significant moral difference because in both cases the anticipated consequence is the same - the death of the patient (the "consequentialists"). On the other hand, others argue it is never morally permissible to take direct action to cause death (the "deontologists"). Which position is correct does not matter in the discussion of aid in dying because this historic debate does not apply.

With aid in dying what is the action of the physician? Is it the action of the physician which causes the patient's death? It is not. After the physician has provided knowledge and a prescription for drugs, the physician must leave the outcome to the patient. The patient may not choose to fill the prescription. Even if the prescription is filled, the patient may choose not to take the drugs. Suppose the patient eventually chooses to take the lethal drugs and dies. In that case, did the doctor do nothing and simply allow the death? Or, did the doctor do something and cause the death?

In legal terms the patient's action is an independent intervening cause. That is, the willful action of the patient after leaving the physician's office is independent of the action of the physician and intervenes to cause the death. This is why a physician assisting a patient in such a way would not be charged with murder even in those jurisdictions where aid in dying is yet prohibited. Murder requires a direct act of killing. With aid in dying it is the patient who independently acts to cause his own death. The doctor simply does not kill the patient.

Assisted death is on the middle ground in the active/passive debate. It is not doing nothing in the face of suffering and a patient's request and it is not acting to cause the death. It is assisting a dying patient at the patient's request and leaving the decision to the patient. It may be because aid in dying is on the middle ground that it is approved by most of us.

2. Intent To Relieve Suffering or Cause Death?

The second historical debate involves the intent of the physician. A distinction is drawn between intending to relieve pain and suffering on the one hand and intending to cause death on the other. This is the doctrine of "double effect."

The AMA agrees that it is morally permissible for a physician to attempt to relieve a patient's suffering *even though* the physician knows the attempt may hasten the death. The physician may ethically prescribe powerful pain medications even with the knowledge that the drug may depress respiration to the point of causing the patient's death. After all, it is not the intent of the physician that the patient die. The death is just the unfortunate and unintended side effect of the well meaning intent to relieve the patient's suffering. What is prohibited is giving the patient drugs with the intent to cause death.

This historic argument also does not apply to aid in dying. What is the intent of the physician in providing aid in dying? The dying patient inquires about hastening death. A process follows and the physician may provide knowledge and a prescription. From that point on the patient may either fill the prescription or not. If the patient fills the prescription then the patient must yet choose whether or not to take the drugs.

Suppose the patient eventually chooses to take the lethal drugs and dies. What was the intent of the physician when providing assistance? Did the physician intend the death of the patient? Or, did the doctor intend for the patient to continue living? It cannot be both. But it can be neither.

The physician's intent is to respect the patient's autonomy and to relieve the patient's suffering and the physician cannot intend or do anything more. The physician cannot intend to cause the death because the physician cannot cause the death. If the intent of the physician is anything it is similar to the intent of the physician who seeks to relieve the patient's suffering *even though* the drugs may cause the death. With aid in dying the intent of the physician is to relieve suffering *even though* the patient may decide in the future to cause her own death.

Even if one or both of these historic distinctions did apply, we could not conclusively determine whether the physician's assistance is right or wrong. Both sides in both debates have proponents advancing subtle and nuanced positions. Who is right in those debates? Again, we must recognize our diversity and uncertainty.

We might also explore the feelings and beliefs of the proponents of each view. What values are you relying upon to support your position? Do your values reflect ultimate truth? May others have different values which should also be respected even if you think they are wrong and tragic?

B.   Is Aid In Dying Contrary to the Goals of Medicine?

Is aid in dying contrary to the goals of medicine? The AMA declares this to be true. But is it true?

Why do physicians do what they do? What do physicians "stand for?" One would hope that all persons would pause to consider the questions: "What is my goal in doing X?" "What is my purpose?"

If the physician has not carefully considered his or her goals in practicing medicine, then the physician cannot possibly reach a proper conclusion regarding whether or not aid in dying is contrary to those goals. The term "goal" simply means the "purpose" or "why" of practice. The physician ought to be able to say, "My goal(s) or purpose(s) in practicing medicine is/are to do X."

What might be considered the goals of medical practice? Consider the following possible answers:

- To treat illness and injury
- To heal (to cure)

- To do no harm
- To do good
- To save lives
- To relieve suffering
- To obey the law
- To respect patient autonomy
- To be medically competent
- To earn money

This list is, no doubt, not all inclusive. It does, however, seem a fair listing of the possible answers to the question. If additional answers come to mind they can be added to this list and analyzed as below.

These goals are not mutually exclusive. In most instances the physician acts in compliance with all or most of these goals. For example, the physician treats in the attempt to cure a disease which will save the patient's life. At the same time the physician cares for and respects the patient, acts competently, does no harm, relieves the patient's suffering, and acts in accordance with the law. The physician is paid for the treatment and, thus, earns a living while fulfilling these other goals.

The ethical dilemmas of medical practice do not arise until these goals and purposes conflict. With aid in dying several conflicts appear to exist. The physician cannot save the life, relieve the suffering, respect the patient's autonomy and obey the law at the same time.

Are any of these goals of medicine of greater value or "primary" to the other stated goals? If it is concluded that a particular goal is primary, it may be that physician assistance in death is compatible with that primary goal and, thus, a proper role of the physician. Can we define the "primary goal" of medical practice? If we must choose but one of the ten candidates as a summary statement of the "fundamental purpose of the practice of medicine" which would we choose?

Several of the possible answers match up with the four principles of bioethics discussed in Part Two. They include the principles of autonomy (to respect patient autonomy), nonmaleficence (to do no harm), benefi-cence (to do good), and justice (to be just). Is the primary goal of medicine simply one of the well known principles of bioethics?

How do we determine which of the stated goals is primary, if any? One way is to seek the goal which requires no further questions of us. For example, and on a broader scale, suppose we wish to know what it is another person wants - primarily wants. We ask the person. He might reply that he wants health, or money, or fame, or children. Obviously, many different answers may be given to the question.

With almost any answer we can continue to respond with the further question: But why? Why do you want money? Because I can buy a house. But why do you want a house? Because I want my own garden. But why do you want a garden? And so on until the person is driven to the answer: "Because it will make me happy." At that point, we would need ask: "But why do you want to be happy?"

In the context of our experience as human beings, however, this is a nonsense question. That is, it seems silly to ask a person why he wants to be happy. The desirability of a "state of happiness" seems self-evident to us. We might ask him why he thinks fame or children or a garden will make him happy, but we do not need to ask why he wants to be happy. *Primarily*, he wants to be happy. That answer needs no further explana-tion. We understand.

In a similar manner we can attempt to define the primary goal of the medical profession. Which of our stated goals, if any, requires no fur-ther questions? Which answer, if stated to be the primary goal of medical practice, needs no further explanation?

Upon examination, the above list of ten primary goal candidates can be separated into four general categories. Some can quickly be desig-nated as "ancillary" or secondary goals of medicine. One of the candi-dates, while it may be the primary goal of some physicians, is also quickly rejected. The third group, while appearing at first to be good candidates for "primary goal," actually constitute what medical practice is, and not what medical practice strives for. Finally, several of the candidates seem actually in the running for the label "primary goal" or "fundamental purpose" of medical practice.

Ancillary Goals - Several of the above candidates can be eliminated fairly easily. Of the original list of ten, three can be labeled no more than ancillary goals. These goals of the physician are real, but they do not constitute the primary purpose of the practice of medicine. Those three are:

- to do no harm
- to be medically competent
- to obey the law

It would be quite unusual for a physician to state that any one of these was the primary goal or purpose of his or her practice. For example, does the physician practice medicine for the purpose of "doing no harm." While this is most certainly a goal of the physician, we would not expect a physician to state: "I practice medicine for the purpose of doing no harm."

The second goal, "to be medically competent," also fits into this category. While a commendable goal, one would not expect a doctor to state that the primary reason she practices medicine is "to be medically competent."

The primary goal of medical practice is also not "to obey the law." Again, one would not hear a physician state that his primary reason for entering medical practice is to obey the law. Obeying the law is a proper and important goal of the physician but it simply cannot be considered the first and foremost reason for medical practice. (In most states physicians pursue this goal by denying their dying patients assistance in death.)

To Earn Money - Next, consider the candidate "to earn money." As before, we would not expect to hear a physician give such an answer. But we might. If the primary reason a physician practices medicine is to earn money, then the physician has made considerations other than money, including the patient, secondary. This discussion will be of little interest to this doctor. Such a physician would not hesitate to assist a patient in death - if he got paid to do so.

To Treat Illness and Injury, To Cure (To Heal) - Many physicians might very well state that the primary goals of their practice are to treat illness and injury and to cure disease. We would not criticize a physician for giving such answers.

Basically, "treating illness and injury" and "curing disease" are, themselves, the practice of medicine. The physician practices. She treats and, hopefully, cures. Treating and curing are the means by which the physician helps the patient. Treating is what the physician does and not why she does it. The physician, *in order to* improve lives, restore autonomy, save lives or relieve suffering, acts to treat illness and cure disease. In other terms, the physician treats and cures *for the purpose of* improving, saving, restoring or relieving. It would yet be proper to ask a physician why she treats illness or why she attempts to cure disease.

Let us note another goal variation here. The goal of the physician is "to heal." This goal is specifically included in light of the position of the AMA. The AMA states that aid in dying "is fundamentally incompatible with the physician's role as healer."

One could argue the definition of the terms "heal" and "healer." In this context, however, a "healer" is one who cures. She "makes well" or restores the patient to health. But we can yet ask why the physician seeks to heal patients. Just as with "treating" and "curing," the physician seeks to heal for the purpose of improving or saving life or relieving suffering.

The candidates from the original list are narrowing. From that list we are now focused upon four possible candidates for the primary goal of medicine. The remaining candidates are - to respect patient autonomy, to save lives, to do good, and to relieve suffering. And this, of course, is precisely where the dilemma of aid in dying resides.

When confronting a dying patient's request to hasten death the physician cannot save the patient's life, honor the patient's choice and relieve the patient's suffering. And we yet do not know if assisting a dying patient is a "good" or a "harm."

To Respect Patient Autonomy - While very important to medical ethics, respecting a patient's autonomy simply is not the primary reason a physician practices medicine. We touch upon the concept of autonomy many times in this discussion and this is one of those topics upon which we could write a book (many have).

We will jump to a conclusion. If "respecting patient autonomy" is the primary purpose of medicine, there would be no objection to assisting the dying individual in death and aid in dying would not be declared contrary to medical ethics.

To Save Lives - There are several reasons why "saving lives" cannot be considered the primary goal of medicine. Most activities which constitute medical practice do not involve "saving lives," whatever that term means. Thousands of doctors treat million of injuries and ailments only a small fraction of which involve "life saving." Far too little of medical practice is concerned with life saving for us to consider "saving lives" to be the primary goal of the medical profession.

Additionally, although saving lives seems obviously important, we can yet ask: Why do physicians seek to save lives? Just why does the physician use all of his or her skill and energy to maintain the life of the patient? Is this a nonsense question, similar to asking a person why he wants to be happy? Is the answer self-evident, needing no further explanation?

Obviously not. This entire discussion is occasioned by the fact that, in some cases, we sincerely question if it is right to insist that dying patients continue their lives. And we question the goal of "saving lives" because they have told us they prefer death to continued dying.

Concentrate on our primary subject again. **DEATH.** Physicians seek to save lives and prevent death *because* death causes fear and loss - suffering. We fight death because we both understand the concept of death and contemplate our own deaths and the deaths of those we love. We do not wish to "suffer" death. If death and the contemplation of death did not cause fear and suffering, our own and others, death would not be fought as it is. There would also be no debates concerning aid in dying.

It is the suffering caused by our anticipated death which makes the prevention of death a major goal of medicine. Physicians practice medicine. They treat and cure and save lives. They do so *because* the treating, curing and saving relieve human suffering.

Although it appears that assisted death creates a conflict between the goal of saving lives and the goals of respecting patient autonomy and relieving patient suffering, no conflict exists. It is important to remember the physician *cannot* save the life of the patient. She cannot, by medical intervention, prevent the impending death. She cannot treat and cure and heal. The patient is dying. This is a premise. Since the goal can no longer be to save the patient's life through medical intervention there is, in fact, no conflict between the goals of "saving life" and "relieving suffering." When one goal can no longer be rationally pursued, one would think the other goal would prevail.

To Do Good - This goal sounds close. One can well imagine a physician declaring that their primary goal is "to do good." After all, "to do good" or "beneficence" is one of the four principles of bioethics. We might all agree that this is the foundational reason for the existence of medicine. Most of us would not think to ask: "Why does the field of medicine want to do good?"

This stated goal is very general. "To do good" could be said to be the goal of many professions. It does seem, however, to encompass the last primary goal candidate which more specifically refers to medical practice. That goal involves the relief of human suffering.

Relief of Suffering is Primary - Our focus does not permit a full discussion of the concept of suffering. We know that human suffering takes many forms. Suffering is often associated with physical pain. Individual suffering may exist in the absence of physical pain, however, and one may not be suffering in the presence of pain. For example, the person who breaks a limb is in pain and is suffering as a result of the physical pain.

On the other hand, a person receiving a tattoo may be in physical pain but deny that he is suffering. Or, he may assert that he is suffering but that "it's worth it." Similarly, a person receiving painful medical treatment may have this attitude. In fact, because the treatment is perceived as healing, the increase in physical pain as a result of the treatment may actually decrease the patient's suffering.

Finally, a person may be in no immediate physical pain but suffering terribly. There is suffering caused by fear, depression, loss, or contemplation of future pain or loss. Obviously, human suffering comes in many different forms.

The suffering caused by or attributed to injury or illness is the suffering we take to the physician. It may be the suffering caused by present physical pain, injury or illness or it may be the suffering generated by the contemplation of future pain, injury or disease.

While not all actions of the physician are directed toward "saving lives," all actions of the physician are aimed at relieving suffering. Physicians examine, diagnose, treat, prescribe, perform surgery and recommend the gamut of clinical possibilities for the express purpose of relieving the patient's suffering. While the physician seeks to do good, the good he seeks is the relief of human suffering.

From the patient's point of view (a most important point of view), the relief of the patient's suffering is not only a goal of the physician but it should be the *only* goal of the physician. Fundamentally, the goal of the patient/physician team is to relieve the patient's suffering.

We can properly add to the definition of this primary goal. The primary purpose of medicine is the relief of human suffering by the application of medical knowledge, techniques and procedures. The physician can, to some extent or completely, by the competent application of clinical skills, technology, procedures and medicines, relieve the pain and suffering caused by the injury, illness or disease. Additionally, with compassion, the physician can offer relief from suffering beyond the physical pain of injury. In this latter role the physician plays the same important function as any other caring person who offers support to the suffering individual.

Of all the candidates for "primary goal" or "purpose" of medicine, "to relieve human suffering" comes closest to being *the* goal, *the* primary purpose, or *the* fundamental reason for the practice of medicine. We ask: What does medicine really want? The ultimate answer is "to relieve human suffering." The answer "to relieve suffering" is very similar to the answer: "I want to be happy." We do not need to ask someone why they want to be happy and we do not need to ask the medical profession why it wants to relieve human suffering. We know why. We understand.

Our understanding is founded in the concept of compassion. Compassion deserves some mention when considering the practice of medicine, aid in dying, or any other area of bioethical concern. Compassion is recognizing and understanding the suffering of others accompanied by the desire to relieve that suffering. Acts of compassion and mercy are acts we recognize as virtuous. It is not surprising that many persons become physicians out of compassion and for the purpose of relieving human suffering. The practice of medicine itself is founded upon this concept.

C.   An Exception to the Goals of Medicine

When individual physicians and the AMA declare it is wrong for a doctor to assist a death they are not making statements which relate to either the primary goal of medicine or any goal of medicine. They are simply declaring a rule of conduct based upon individual perception of right and wrong action. Physicians do this often.

- "I will not perform an abortion. It is sinful."
- "I will not prescribe birth control. It is immoral."
- "I will not assist the dying to die. It is wrong."

A declaration that doctors must not provide aid in dying is, in fact, an *exception* to the goals of medicine.

Some physicians believe the primary purpose of medicine is to relieve human suffering - *except* when it involves assistance in death. Some doctors believe a major goal of medicine is to respect patient autonomy - *except* when it involves aid in dying. Some physicians choose not to relieve suffering or respect their patient's autonomy if it means assisting a dying person in death.

D. Physician Objection is Permitted

Regardless of the goals of medicine, physicians may yet respond to a request for assistance in death by stating: "I just can't do it." It is proper, that is, if the physician's refusal is based upon individual feelings or personal beliefs. Some physicians simply feel or believe so strongly they cannot bring themselves to participate in patient deaths.

We allow individuals to refrain from activities contrary to their strongly held convictions. We should allow the physician the same right without condemnation. There is room in medicine for physicians who cannot do everything. Let them do what they can. But the physician who opposes aid in dying should not assert that the physician who will assist the dying patient is acting contrary to the proper goals of medicine and should be jailed.

E. Do We Need Physicians To Participate?

Do we need physicians to assist dying patients in death? Not necessarily.

It is obvious why those facing death look to physicians for assistance. Physicians tend the sick and the dying. Dying individuals who seek to hasten death seek the easiest method of doing so. They seek a quick and pain-less death. Such a death seems to involve a combination of deadly drugs. Physicians have knowledge of drugs and we have given physicians the power to prescribe. It is also the security of the important physician/patient relationship we rely upon to help insure that patients are not mistreated.

It is certainly true, however, that others could fulfill this function. Pharmacists know about drugs. Hospice organizations provide support to dying patients who wait for death. Others could be trained to assist these few patients.

At the same time, however, many physicians do not object to this role. Here it is simply recognized that others could properly perform this function. Until there is a substantial change in societal roles, however, physicians will be the ones the dying look to for assistance to the end.

F.   The Physician's Position

If one accepts the premises that (1) the primary goal or medicine is to relieve human suffering, (2) that goal flows from the concept of compassion, (3) compassion and the relief of suffering are virtues, and (4) death is not the worst thing that can happen to dying patients, then assisting a dying, suffering patient in death is not contrary to the goals of medicine and should not be considered contrary to medical ethics. The conclusions follow from the premises.

The physician may take several positions regarding aid in dying. The physician who accepts the above conclusions might state to his patient:

> "You sought me out to help relieve the suffering caused by your condition. I have used my knowledge and skills as best I could to treat you and extend your life. I acted in accordance with the primary goal of my profession. You are now dying. I cannot save you. It is your decision to hasten your death rather than prolong the dying process. You ask for my help to die in a quick and painless way. I will not abandon you. My medical knowledge can yet be used to help you. I will assist you to manage your death in accordance with your competent wishes. It will be my last act as your physician to relieve your suffering."

On the other hand, the physician may still maintain the position that his or her participation is wrong. The continued objection may be the result of strongly held feelings or religious beliefs. What are these physicians really saying to their patients?

> ". . . You are now dying. I cannot save you. It is your decision to hasten your death rather than prolong the dying process. You ask for my help. I cannot help you. Although it is your competent decision, I feel and/or believe too strongly about this and my personal feelings/beliefs must prevail."

Physicians who refuse to assist the dying patient because they think the AMA has it right are, in reality, saying the following to the patient (and there is no easy way to say this).

> ". . . I cannot help you. Regardless of your impending death, your suffering, and your considered request, in your case the fundamental goals of relieving suffering and respecting your competent decisions no longer apply. We think your prolonged dying to be better professional and public policy."

Physicians are diverse. They feel and believe differently. They perceive their ethical responsibilities differently. Most will admit to uncertainty concerning what is ultimately true, good, bad, right and wrong.

Some physicians have feelings, beliefs or values which cause them to oppose aid in dying. Many physicians do not. The fact that some do, however, cannot justify the use of force against those who do not.

Part Four

Will Aid In Dying Cause More Harm Than Good?

Even if it is not wrong for a dying individual to hasten death with the assistance of a physician, should aid in dying yet be prohibited because it will cause more harm than good?

Here is where we find most of the continuing opposition.

There has been no shortage of individuals and organizations predicting that aid in dying will cause terrible consequences for patients, medicine, and society. The American Medical Association joined those with such visions when declaring in 1994 (and still declaring) that aid in dying would "be difficult or impossible to control and would pose serious societal risks."

These arguments were widely employed and quite effective twenty years ago. Because they involved fears, speculation and predictions of future behavior they were impossible to rebut. How could one disprove future visions? But one must ask some very relevant and obvious questions today. Why are they still being raised? Why would anyone rely upon speculation instead of known experience? Why haven't the arguments based upon those false predictions been neutralized by now? At this point and with over twenty years experience in Oregon and Washington one might simply declare:

> "Thank you for giving this considerable thought and the warnings but your visions were not accurate. The

Oregon and Washington laws are working as intended. We took your fears and speculation into consideration and designed procedures and safeguards to guard against those possible harms. It is quite controlled and limited while allowing for individual freedom in this most personal decision. In fact, it has presented society with no new risks."

As evidenced in every debate, however, such a reasonable response has not satisfied those who continue to oppose aid in dying. And it is not thought that two or three (or ten) more decades of failed predictions will halt their opposition. After all, fundamental feelings and beliefs are at stake. It is certainly true that some religious groups, constrained or reluctant to argue religious doctrine, seek to generate fear with continued predictions of terrible harms.

While our experience alone should put these arguments to rest, these "consequence" arguments are also without ethical basis to justify the criminalization of aid in dying.

A. "Consequence" Arguments Are Not Arguments Against Aid In Dying Itself

In Part 2 we briefly discussed utilitarian ethical theories which focus on the consequences of actions. Those theories tell us the right conduct is that which brings about more good than harm. Let us adopt the utilitarian view. Let us agree if the consequences of permitting aid in dying are more harmful than beneficial, to individuals or society, aid in dying is bad public policy and can be properly prohibited.

It is important to note that "consequence" arguments tell us nothing about the rightness or wrongness of aid in dying itself. There are opponents who would admit this is true and permit such assistance if it could be limited to the few cases where it properly applies. They do not declare the act of the dying individual to hasten death to be morally wrong. They insist, however, it cannot be properly limited and will cause social harm. There will be unintended bad consequences along with the intended good results. It is because it will lead to terrible harms it should be prohibited.

Consequence arguments against assisted death can be divided into two categories. First, aid in dying cannot be properly managed and policed. Permitting this practice will lead to terrible harms even in the attempt "to do it right." Second, if aid in dying is permitted it will place us upon the infamous "slippery slope." Other terrible practices are certain to follow if we permit such deaths.

There are several significant reasons why these arguments fail. First, aid in dying does not present society with any new risks. Second, we can design safeguards to prevent harmful consequences. Third, the predictions have been wrong. Fourth, some of the the predicted dangers, if they do appear, will appear regardless of whether aid in dying is permitted or prohibited. Finally, and importantly, aid in dying should be seen as *protection* from those feared consequences.

B.   Aid in Dying Cannot be Properly Managed and Policed

Should aid in dying remain illegal because it cannot be properly managed and policed?

These concerns focus upon the patient's state of mind and medical condition and the evil intent of others. Patients may be coerced. They may be severely depressed. They may be irrationally suicidal. Physicians may make mistakes. Consider each of these predicted harms and why the arguments fail.

1.   Coercion

The continuing argument is, if a dying person is permitted to hasten death, then patients will be coerced to end their lives. This pressure may come from families, heirs, doctors, insurance companies or the government. Or, it may come from within. We hear arguments similar to these.

> "We cannot allow aid in dying because patients will be pressured or coerced by others to kill themselves."

> "We must protect vulnerable people from possible pressure from families, heirs, doctors, insurance companies, and government agents."

> "There is a legitimate state interest in protecting vulnerable people from pressure to consent to their own killing."

We will spend more time analyzing this argument because the nature, the reasons for, the problems with, and the result will be the same for a number of the following predicted harmful consequences.

Inconsistency - We will assume this speculation is true. We will assume there may be family members or heirs or others who want the dying patient dead! While this is an extraordinary assumption, we will make it for purposes of this argument. Does this possibility create a new risk for individuals and is it a sufficient reason for prohibition?

Here is the principle involving coercion which is being used to justify the criminalization of aid in dying:

> It is wrong for a person to be coerced into making the choice to hasten death. It is possible that a dying patient may be coerced into making that choice. Because this is true, the choice should always be prohibited.

Do you stand by this principle? If you do then you should understand and appreciate the many other cases which occur far more frequently in medicine and which present even a higher risk of coercion.

These cases involve patients who either refuse life saving medical treatment or withdraw from life saving medical treatment. Many different examples could be given but we only need two simple cases to make this point.

Some patients need life saving blood transfusions. A future patient may have family members who want him dead and who bring pressure upon the patient to refuse the transfusion. The patient may succumb to the pressure and refuse and die.

Some patients are being maintained by dialysis. The dialysis is time consuming and inconvenient but life saving. A patient may have heirs who want the patient to die. They may coerce the patient to withdraw from treatment. She may give in to that pressure, withdraw from dialysis, and die.

In the context of the argument of coercion, what is the difference between the dying patient and these two patients who are not dying? There is none.

The patient refusing the life saving transfusion has a choice between different courses of action (one of which will bring death). It is possible the patient may be coerced into choosing the course which brings death. Because of the possibility of coercion, should the choice be prohibited? Who is willing to make the argument that, *because of the possibility of coercion*, no patient should ever be allowed to refuse blood transfusions or any other life saving medical treatment?

It is the same for the dialysis patient. It is possible the patient may be vulnerable and coerced by greedy heirs into refusing further dialysis and dying. Should we prohibit the choice? Again, is there anyone, including theologians or bioethicists, who will argue that the choice to withdraw from life saving medical treatment should be prohibited because of some future possibility of patient coercion?

In fact, the possibility of coercion in refusal and withdrawal cases is most certainly higher than with aid in dying. With aid in dying the patient is terminal. It will not be long before those greedy families achieve their objective - a dead relative. Only a little patience is required.

On the other hand, in cases involving refusal or withdrawal from life saving treatment the patient is not dying. It may be years or decades before their death would be expected. More than a little patience would be required of those deadly families. They have a real motive to coerce their family member to exercise the legal choice of death.

Internal Pressure - There is also the fear that dying patients may place pressure upon themselves. Some will argue along these lines:

> "If the patient is at home, many frustrations and demands may be imposed on the family by the illness. The patient may have extreme weakness, incontinence, and bad odors. The pressure of caring for the dying person under these circumstances is likely to cause a resentment on the part of those who have to do the nursing and guilt on the part of the patient."

> "Is this the kind of choice we want to offer a dying person? Will we not also sweep up those who are not really tired of life, but think others are tired of them, those who do not really want to die, but who feel they should not live on."

Not only can one be coerced by others, but one can also be pressured by feelings, beliefs, or other considerations. This is a difficult area to resolve and a volume could be dedicated to what it means to make a "free choice" and when free choice is extinguished by internal pressures. Is the faithful Jehovah's Witness "pressured" by her religious beliefs?

What can we say about the patient who is dying and is thinking: "I am dying and a burden and I will bankrupt my family if I continue to receive these expensive medical treatments." We can assume these thoughts enter the minds of some dying individuals.

We cannot know everything the dying patient might be considering. We can ask them. They may or may not be honest with us. But what is a proper consideration for a dying individual and what is not? What do we say to the individual if we refuse their choice based upon our belief they "felt internal pressure?"

We can tell them they should not feel guilt. We can instruct them they should not believe as they do. We can state they should not be considering those things. We can offer comfort and support. There are many things we can do.

If they express these feelings we can even argue with them (appropriately and without coercion). We can try to change their view and assure them they are not a burden or that "it will be alright." But if in the end we cannot eliminate their feelings or beliefs or their consideration of consequences and their conclusions, what are we to do? Do we forbid everyone from making a choice because we think some individuals feel or believe or might be considering things we do not think they should feel or believe or need to be considering?

We should be concerned about coercion involving life and death medical decisions but it should be equal concern in all cases. In each of these situations there is medical distress. The patient is dying or may die. The choice is the same - between a course of action which continues life or a course which hastens death. The possibility of pressure and coercion (from outside or within) is equal. The result of the coerced choice is the same - death. Although the identical concepts and fears apply in refusal and withdrawal cases, no one is suggesting that the choices of all patients be limited because of possible cases of coercion. And we will not. We should not.

Since this is the case, we must ask if the coercion argument made in opposition to aid in dying is an honest argument. Is it a consistent concern? Is it a real concern regarding patient coercion if the concern is not being similarly shown in similar cases? Or, is the argument advanced against aid in dying simply by those who, for whatever reasons, oppose aid in dying?

Safeguards - We can demonstrate a very different outcome regarding the possibility of coercion where aid in dying is permitted. Permitting assisted death *protects* vulnerable patients from coercion.

Deadly and uncaring families will exist whether aid in dying is permitted or not. Where it is prohibited those families can bully the patient behind closed doors. They can pressure the dying person to "get it over with" without outside interference. After all, you don't need a physician to die.

Where aid in dying is permitted legal safeguards are in place and others are involved. There is a system and procedures to ensure a voluntary request by a competent, adult patient under the care of physicians. (It is worth noting that none of these specific statutory procedures and safeguards apply to patients who choose to die by refusing or withdrawing from life saving medical treatment.)

The wishes of the patient are in the open and subject to the judgment of other disinterested persons and professionals. There is opportunity to test the patient's desires and to weigh other possible options involving pain, suffering and support. There is opportunity to intervene in troubling cases.

Experience - The fear of coercion was recognized and legal safeguards were placed in the Oregon law. With over a decade and a half of experience, no evidence exists that patients are being coercion into "choosing" aid in dying. Experience trumps speculation.

What if Coercion Does Occur? - Suppose we do have evidence that a family is pressuring a patient to hasten death. This concern applies equally to all cases of life saving medical treatment. What should be our reaction?

Obviously, if we have a hint of pressure or coercion during the process of decision making extra caution should be taken to ascertain the competency and wishes of the patient.

If the evidence of family pressure or coercion surfaces after the choice and after the death, it is difficult to know what to say. The State of Oregon makes it a felony to coerce a patient. "A person who coerces or exerts undue influence on a patient to request medication for the purpose of ending the patient's life, or to destroy a rescission of such a request, shall be guilty of a Class A felony." (ORS 127.890 §4.02)

In Oregon evidence can be given to the local prosecutor. But the fact that it might occur in any of these cases adds nothing to the argument that we should prohibit everyone from making the choice because it might happen again.

What else can we do to eliminate this speculated harm and the use of fear in the public debates? Let the social scientists go to work. Let them study all cases equally and make honest findings regarding the possibility of coercion. Is this a realistic concern? Is it an honest reason for the continued criminalization of aid in dying? Unless and until fair studies can be conducted comparing assisted death cases with refusal and withdrawal cases to demonstrate that others are more apt to pressure or coerce terminally ill patients, the coercion arguments should be given no weight.

In all cases we should have equal concern for the patient and make equal inquiry relating to the patient's circumstance, competence and choice. No more, no less. There is simply no reason in logic, medical ethics or law why the possibility of coercion should apply differently in cases of aid in dying.

2. Depressed or Suicidal Persons

There is much opposition to aid in dying based upon the fear that a dying patient may be severely depressed or "suicidal."

The principle here is similar. It is possible that a dying patient may be depressed or suicidal. Because this is true, the choice should always be prohibited.

We will assume that "clinically depressed" (however it is defined) and "suicidal" persons are not competent to make the life and death decision we are concerned with.

We can assume that terminally ill persons are depressed. We can suppose that they are not elated or happy in any significant way. But does an unhappy or depressed person equal an incompetent person? Are they necessarily robbed of the ability to make a rational choice? Should we deny them their autonomy?

This argument also applies a double standard and is inconsistently applied.

Who is a "competent" person? Much has been written regarding the concept of competency. We will limit the discussion to two relevant points. First, we know how to make determinations of competency. Second, and again, there is no reason to direct this concern solely toward those who seek aid in dying.

We must determine the competency (or capacity) of all patients making medical treatment decisions and especially patients facing life and death decisions. When we are making determinations of a patient's competency we are, in effect, asking one question: Should we allow this person to make this decision at this time and under these circumstances?

Patients should be determined competent if (1) they have an understanding of the situation, (2) they understand the options and the consequences of the decision, and (3) they give rational reasons for their decision. In all cases, if patients meet the above criteria, we should consider them "competent" and respect the choice. In all cases, if the patient fails one of these important criteria, we should consider them incompetent and not allow them to decide. Sometimes it is quite easy to make determinations of competency and sometimes it is quite difficult. But we must always make this attempt. We are able to conduct the investigation of a patient's competency in cases of assisted death as well as in cases of refusal and withdrawal and we should do so.

Inconsistency - Just as with opposition based upon coercion, one must ask why this argument is aimed solely at aid in dying. The situation is identical to refusal and withdrawal cases. A patient is in medical distress and has a choice. The choice is whether to take action which will hasten the death or not. The ethical concepts are identical. Is the patient competent to make this decision or not? The legal conclusions should be identical. Opposition to aid in dying based upon the possibility of depressed, suicidal or incompetent patients fails the consistency test. It is not applied equitably. It does not appear honestly made.

Safeguards - We already know we must determine the competency of individuals making life and death decisions and we already know how to make these determinations. In Oregon safeguards are specifically included within the statute to ensure this process takes place properly. And, again, no such extra precautions are in place for those who will die because they refuse or withdraw from life extending treatments.

Experience - With over twenty years experience there exists no evidence that incompetent patients are being allowed to "choose" aid in dying in Oregon and Washington. Experience trumps speculation.

3. Medical Mistakes

What if the diagnosis and/or the prognosis is wrong? What if the patient is not really dying? We often hear:

> "It is impossible for any physician to know if a patient is going to die within six months. Doctors are fallible human beings."

We understand this concern. We know that physicians make mistakes. They are not infallible. The physician may be wrong regarding the terminal condition or when the patient is expected to die. Is this a justification for prohibiting aid in dying?

What is the principal involved with opposition based upon possible mistakes? It is similar to the coercion reasoning. Something bad might happen. Because a medical mistake may occur in a future case(s) no patient should ever be allowed the choice of aid in dying. And similar to coercion, should we forbid everyone at all times and under all circumstances from making choices because in some future case(s) a mistake may be made?

These are situations where competent adults must be allowed to exercise their judgment. Such personal decisions require personal judgments.

"What is my medical history? What do I know? What have I been told? How do I feel? How is my pain? Do I trust my physicians? Do I have hope? Is continued treatment beneficial or futile? Can I expect a miracle? Is my doctor wrong? Am I afraid of death? Can I go on? Do I want to prolong my dying? Is my death worse than my continued dying?"

What kinds of decisions are these? They are not medical decisions to be made by the physician or the AMA. They are not legal decisions to be made by lawyers or judges. They are not social decisions to be made by a majority. They are extremely personal decisions.

Safeguards - We will never be able to eliminate all medical errors. If we prohibit choices because doctors sometimes make mistakes we will bring the field of medicine to a halt. In all of medicine we can take steps to reduce those possible errors and safeguard patients.

The fear of physician mistake was recognized and addressed in the Oregon statute which requires the involvement of multiple physicians.

In all cases and at all times, if there are other reasonable means of preventing medical mistakes, then they should be proposed. The possibility of physician error, however, simply cannot be used to justify the use of force against those who choose to participate in aid in dying.

Experience - With over twenty years experience there is no evidence that physicians are making diagnostic or prognostic mistakes which lead patients to mistakingly choose aid in dying. Experience trumps speculation.

4. Eliminate the Pain

We hear arguments involving patient pain.

"Dying patients should not be suffering from pain. If they had adequate pain relief they would not be asking for aid in dying. Thus, we should prohibit all dying patients from choosing to hasten death and simply do more to relieve their pain."

Debilitating pain can be a major factor at the end of life. We will assume it is true that pain relief will extinguish the desire to hasten death for many if not most persons. We agree that everyone should do everything at all times to reduce every patient's pain. We are in agreement. Now what do we do in the few cases where the relief is not sufficient or, in spite of sufficient physical pain relief, other factors drive the patient's choice?

5. Not Sufficient Suffering

Opposition to the Oregon statute is even based upon the fact that the Oregon law does not specifically require "suffering" as a necessary condition to a request. The principle here, it is supposed, is that if we are going to allow dying patients to hasten death, then we should make absolutely certain that they are *really* in pain and/or *really* suffering.

First, we do not require any suffering, much less extraordinary suffering, of patients who are not dying but who choose death by refusing or withdrawing from life saving treatment. Individuals who are expected to live for years if not decades are allowed to choose death. If they are competent it is their decision without any "degree of suffering" requirement.

Second, as discussed in Part Three, human suffering can take many forms. It may be physical or mental. It may be more or less from moment to moment. We can ask a patient if they are suffering but would that be sufficient?

If lack of a "suffering" requirement in the law is the reason for opposing aid in dying we should simply ask those who demand a requirement of suffering to draft the definition they would prefer. Once we have language drafted we can discuss how it would be applied. It is thought that it would be considerably more difficult to determine whether or not a dying patient has met the "degree of extraordinary suffering" requirement than to determine whether or not a patient is competent.

6. Harm to Families

Opponents argue that aid in dying will cause harm to families. Because this is true, no one should ever be allowed to make this choice.

We can assume that loving families are hurt by the deaths of their loved ones. (This discussion excludes the deadly families who will coerce their family members to die.) These are difficult circumstances to say the least. The patient is dying. The patient is suffering in one manner or another and to some degree or another. The dying process is difficult for everyone. How can a caring family not be suffering along with the patient?

But after all things are considered, including family relationships, if the patient chooses to hasten his own death, to what additional extent is the family harmed? More basically, whose decision is this? Who is to decide these things? Should family members be allowed to coerce continued life if we will not allow them to coerce death? Are we to legally assume that in all cases at all times families think the death of their dying family member is the worse thing that can happen?

Let the social scientists study families where requests have been made under the Oregon and Washington statutes. Let them study (1) the families of patients who have made requests of their physicians (2) the families of those who filled their prescriptions but did not use them and (3) the families of those who took the final step and used the drugs. Did those families support or oppose the patient's decision? Have they been harmed by the patient's decision?

Of course, to be fair we should have other studies for comparison. They should also study the harm to families of those who were dying and who wished to hasten their own deaths but were prevented by state statute from receiving aid in dying. Has there been harm to those families?

7. Harm to the Physician/Patient Relationship

It is argued if we permit physicians to assist their patients in death, the relationship between physicians and patients will be harmed.

Regardless of such speculation, public opinion evidences that most of us do not think the relationship will be harmed. Most of us think our physicians should be allowed to assist us in this final act. But, again, let the social scientists conduct studies.

Let us inquire in states that allow aid in dying whether there has been a harmful change in the nature of the physician/patient relationship. In Oregon we might ask:

> "Since 1998 has your relationship with your doctor changed? At this time is your relationship worse, better, unchanged? Do you now trust your physician more or less?" And so on.

This does not appear to be a difficult task and it would be useful to put this opposition argument to rest. The findings should certainly be sent to the American Medical Association.

8. Aid in Dying Cannot Be Limited

Some oppose aid in dying because they fear it cannot be limited to the current statutory requirements and we will be forced to confront other difficult cases.

For example, consider a case in which a competent terminally ill patient makes a request for aid in dying pursuant to the Oregon statute. Every step in the process is properly completed. The prescription is written and the lethal drugs are obtained. Then, however, the patient becomes incompetent. If the drugs are consumed and the patient dies, is this a voluntary death or an involuntary death (incompetent persons cannot give a valid consent)? Is it right or is it wrong? Should this death be prohibited or permitted?

Or suppose the patient is yet competent but the patient's physical condition has deteriorated and they can no longer self-administer the drugs. The patient requests final assistance. If someone else assists the patient is this wrong? Should those actions be permitted?

Cases with variation of facts will always arise. We cannot prevent this from happening. Life goes on. Life is change and challenge and uncertainty. New cases will arise which will give us pause.

Some will argue that aid in dying should be permitted in one or both of those cases. You may fear those other cases. But the fact that difficult cases will arise in the future should not diminish our ability to think and reach conclusions today. Neither of those possible cases diminish the arguments for permitting aid in dying.

Some argue if patient autonomy and relief of suffering are the primary values fueling the legalization of aid in dying, there are similar situations in which a person ought to be allowed to choose death. Patients may be in extreme pain or otherwise suffering terribly but not dying. Shouldn't those suffering individuals also be able to choose and receive assistance in hastening their own deaths? How are they different?

Those cases are significantly different because aid in dying concerns the *dying*. This is further discussed in Part 5 where we clarify what aid in dying is really about. It is about managing the deaths of the dying.

The fear of being unable to limit aid in dying is the fear of the "slippery slope." But isn't it better to venture out onto the slope aware of the possible dangers? Knowing our fears and with concern for possible harms we can be cautious and make our way with care. Being stuck on a mountain ledge forever does not appear to be a viable option. ("Slippery slope" concerns are discussed further below.)

9.   What if the Speculated Harms Do Occur?

We do have concerns regarding each of the feared harms. Each is a legitimate concern in each individual case. Is the patient being coerced? Is the patient competent to make such a choice? Has a prognostic mistake been made?

We can guard against those concerns. The State of Oregon places far more statutory safeguards upon aid in dying then other situations involving life and death medical decisions.

It is not sufficient to bring forth a case or an anecdote in which someone did something wrong and then claim "proof" that aid in dying cannot be controlled. If that is a basis for prohibition then surgery and much of medicine will be prohibited. But if experience demonstrates that the safeguards and procedures established in Oregon and other states are not sufficient to alleviate our concerns, then other reasonable procedures can be established in your state. Until that time, however, speculation cannot justify criminalization.

10. Speculated Harm versus Known Benefits

A discussion of possible harm should also include a discussion of the benefits of permitting aid in dying.

We know in states where aid in dying is prohibited there are individuals who are dying and would choose to hasten death. What is their current situation?

These dying individuals have no legal avenue to pursue. They have no knowledge and they cannot discuss options with their physician. Some seek out books on how to end their own lives. Some quietly search for Dr. Kervorkian's successors. Some will eventually choose violent deaths. Guns and automobile "accidents" and other violent acts can also cause harm to families and society. And in rare cases we see "mercy killings." We know that, regardless of legal consequences, some persons take things into their own hands.

These are harms that currently exist with the criminalization of aid in dying. These are harms that are eliminated by society's recognition that they are not just "suicides." This is not speculation about what may occur. These are harms we know can be eliminated.

Here is another possible benefit. Oregon reports that between 1998 through 2012 1,173 individuals sought out their physicians and received prescriptions for the drugs necessary to hasten death. Only 752 patients eventually used the drugs. Did the mere possession and control of the means of death give those who did not consume the drugs the will to go on? Did they receive comfort from the knowledge that they controlled their own fate sufficient to continue living?

Consider also what currently occurs quietly in the dark and without full disclosure in most of the United States. Fear of the dying process and suffering have always existed. We know physicians have always managed the dying process by assisting some patients to die.

It would be interesting to know how many deaths have occurred because doctors have agreed, in one manner or another, to assist the patient and hasten death. We do not know because we criminalize such conduct and no one reports these deaths.

C. Slippery Slopes and the "Culture of Death"

Opponents of aid in dying are worried about much more than uncaring families, suicidal persons and doctors making mistakes. Some opponents predict terrible societal consequences.

One hears numerous arguments opposing aid in dying based upon "slippery slopes." These arguments predict that allowing assistance in death will put us upon a "slippery slope" and we will slide into other, evil actions. We will change our values and our culture and those changes will not be for the good. We will become a "culture of death" in which the deaths of others will not be considered a harm but will be encouraged and promoted. Here are typical examples of "slippery slope" arguments against aid in dying.

> "Aid in dying will lead to a diminished respect for life which will make all of our lives less valuable and we will end up caring less about the elderly and the mentally retarded."

> "I foresee the danger that legal procedures initially designed to permit those who are a nuisance to themselves may someday swallow up those who are a nuisance to others."

"We will declare a 'duty to die' in the hopes of getting the dying out of the way. We will begin the involuntary killing of those who do not meet the rules established for aid in dying. And, finally, society will be so comfortable with the death of others that we will simply begin murdering our fellow citizens - killing the old and disabled."

Once again, these arguments tell us nothing about the ethics or morality of aid in dying itself. They relate to visions. Aid in dying "will lead to . . . ," "may someday . . .", and "we will begin to . . . ."

Slippery slope arguments are very suspect. They do not involve facts. They do not involve actions that are occurring or will immediately occur. They cannot now be disproved. They involve fears and substantial speculation relating to human psychology and future behavior. They do no more than speculate and conclude.

"Aid In dying will lead to the murdering of disabled people. Murdering disabled people is wrong. Thus, aid in dying should be criminal."

The Conceptual Tar Pit - To oppose the slippery slope let us introduce the "conceptual tar pit." A conceptual tar pit is an area where a proper idea cannot escape a pit of bad ideas and horror stories. Regardless of substantial differences involving both action and intent, aid is dying is being tarred by an imagined society that cannot think and does not care. We should also be careful to avoid conceptual tar pits.

Are these predicted fears realistic? Is there a likelihood they will occur? Is there a small chance they will occur? What do we know now that relates to these predicted horrors? What is it that has occurred or is occurring today that makes such a view of the future plausible? Are there other societal changes which are just as likely to occur? What can be done to prevent such evils? What does our experience evidence? What can we do if they do occur?

Byron Chell

Let us extract aid in dying from this tar pit of horror stories. Again, it is better to be aware and cautious on a slippery slope than stuck forever on a mountain ledge or embedded in a tar pit.

The pit contains several different but related fears including the creation of a "duty to die" and murder.

1. Duty to Die

The concern that allowing aid in dying will create a "duty to die" has been heard often. We hear statements like these.

> "It is possible that a social and psychological climate will be created under which dying individuals would be expected to kill themselves."

> "Opening up of the option of assisted suicide will greatly constrain human choice. Choosing death is not one option among many, but an option to end all options. There will be great pressure on the aged and the vulnerable to exercise this option. Once the legal option to hasten death arrives, it will plague and weigh on every decision made by any seriously ill elderly person - not to speak of their more powerful caretakers - even without the subtle hints and pressures applied to them by others."

This speculative argument must also fail because (1) there is no evidence that such a duty has arisen or will arise, and (2) there is alternative speculation which is just as valid.

It is quite easy to imagine a time of limited medical resources. How about the present? We know that a significant amount of our health care resources are spent treating individuals in the last six months of life. We know there are many dying individuals who ask others to do everything, including spending unlimited resources, to prolong their lives for months or weeks or days. Are those persons currently under pressure to die?

This is not the place for an extended discussion regarding how to pay for and allocate our health care resources and the dysfunctional manner in which we continue to deal with these issues. That debate has raged for decades. It did not arise because of assisted death and it will not disappear whether we permit or prohibit aid in dying. But because we have been struggling with this issue for awhile we can ask a number of questions relevant to the concern over aid in dying.

What has been the effect of our societal struggle to date? What is our current experience with dying patients? Is there evidence that today's patients feel a "duty to die" and are encouraged to refuse or withdraw from expensive treatment because we are short of health care resources? Are we now urging patients to forego treatments and die? Have we created the attitude that they do not have a right to those things? Are we insinuating that they have a duty to forego further expensive care and to accept death? Have our societal pressures created a "duty to die?" This has not occurred in Oregon. Why will permitting a small number of persons to hasten death be the action that leads to a "duty to die?"

Predicting that aid in dying will someday lead to a "duty to die" is wonderful in argument because it cannot be disproved. But speculation can go in many directions. Here is a prediction which is just as valid.

Because we know what modern medical technology can do we encourage individuals to complete advance directives. With an advance directive we can set out our desires regarding the use of life support if we are unable to communicate our desires. We can prepare forms that instruct others when attempts to maintain our life should cease. This has been a major effort throughout the country for the past several decades.

Let us speculate and predict.

Advance directives are dangerous and should not be allowed! If we allow this practice to continue our societal values will change. It will be slow but advance directives put us on a slippery slope and they will eventually lead us to terrible evils. The ability to choose to forego life extending efforts will eventually result in a duty to die and murder. You can see how this will happen.

"You *may* fill out an advance directive and instruct that efforts to extend your life should cease if that is your desire." But because of pressures on our medical resources this will lead to the next step.

"You *ought* to fill out an advance directive and instruct that efforts to extend your life should cease if that is your desire." But this will lead to the next step.

"You *must* fill out an advance directive and instruct that efforts to extend your life should cease." And the next step.

"You *do not need* to fill out an advance directive. Your desires no longer matter. There is an obligation on everyone to forego life sustaining procedures. Everyone has a duty to die." Ultimately, of course, because of continuing societal pressures this will lead to final step.

"We simply must eliminate the continuing nuisance, burden and costs associated with health care for the elderly, the vulnerable and the disabled. They should be killed!"

We can speculate that these things will occur. Science fiction writers do it often. We can predict that our society will at some future date create a duty to die and then begin to murder persons because those evil actions will follow from our current desire that patients have advance directives regarding continued life support. After all, such instructions tell us that death can be a preferred option. How is this speculation any less valid than the speculation that allowing competent dying persons the choice to hasten death will lead to the obligation of all dying patients to die?

In reality, and to return to a sensible world, promoting advance directives simply means we wish to emphasize that we have a right to make choices when it comes to death and dying. That is our current societal conclusion involving advance directives.

The ethical issues surrounding aid in dying are, in fact, most similar to the ethical issues surrounding advance directives. Each and every bioethical concept which applies to advance directives applies to aid in dying.

With both advance directives and aid in dying we are involved with life prolonging decisions. In each instance there may be uncertainty regarding what is ultimately right and the proper course of action. With an advance directive we allow you to tell us how we should proceed when it comes to continued life support. With aid in dying we allow you to tell us how you wish to proceed with dying and death. In both instances we emphasize the importance of individual choice.

This attitude regarding individual choice leads to the next important point.

2. Aid in Dying As Protection

Beyond creating a "duty to die," it is argued that the path of aid in dying will lead us to the involuntary killing of vulnerable persons. Here is truly a big picture view. It is not that permitting aid in dying is terrible in itself. It is not that horrible harms will appear immediately. It will be slow. It will be subtle. But allowing assisted death will put our society on the road to destruction. We hear arguments similar to this:

> "If voluntary deaths are legalized, there is good reason to believe that at a later date another bill for mandatory deaths will be legalized. Once the respect for human life is so low that we may kill an innocent person even at his own request, compulsory deaths will necessarily be very close. This could lead easily to killing all incurable charity patients, the aged who are a public care, wounded soldiers, all deformed children, the mentally afflicted, and so on. Before long the danger would be at the door of every citizen."

First, such predictions must be seen for what they are - gross speculation. Why is it predicted that aid in dying will change societal attitudes about death and lessen respect for life? Why isn't it predicted that aid in dying will change our attitudes about personal freedom and increase respect for individual choice?

Death is inevitable. We all know this. Those who support aid in dying also support medical attempts to improve life and prevent death. They do not "love death" and they do not promote death. They do, however, recognize the reality of death. Death is coming, wanted or not. We had better learn how to go about it. Recognizing those things, supporter's seek to give the individual a choice concerning the individual's death. The change in Oregon, Washington and Vermont is a societal change in attitude about personal freedom and liberty, not death.

If you fear a culture of involuntary killing you should not fear a society moving *toward* more individual freedom. Contrary to the fears of some, aid in dying should be seen as a significant protection against a "culture of death." Permitting aid in dying places us further down the road of individual choice and further away from evil government control.

Additionally, aid in dying is simply not on a slope where one can slide from assisted death to murder. One cannot slide from the dying patient who says "I want to hasten my own death" to "we should kill you even though you are not dying and do not want to die." This is not a slide. This is a leap from a large mountain in one state to a peak in a neighboring state. Instead of placing us on a dangerous slope, aid in dying provides protection in a shelter of individual choice and voluntary action.

Arguments involving Nazi behavior frequently enter the debate. But why? With assisted death no one is killing anyone. To the contrary, everyone is allowing a competent dying individual to make their own choice and act on their own. That was not Nazi policy. The Nazi policy was murder. And the murderous actions were not founded upon a history of allowing individual's to make their own decisions in these matters. The murders were state controlled genocide for political purposes. The feelings, beliefs, and reasoning that lead to murder are so vastly different from those involved with aid in dying that it is hard to know where to begin to engage this argument.

If it is truly believed that society may in the future wish to kill the vulnerable, then be on constant guard against demigods, religious zealots, totalitarian rule, and genocide. Be on guard against those who will take away individual liberty, not those who would grant more personal freedom. And because of the enormous differences between permitting individual freedom of choice on the one hand and involuntary killing on the other, it can be confidently predicted that many proponents of aid in dying will be in the front lines opposing anyone who suggests the involuntary killing of the old and disabled.

If our society should reach the point where we willingly begin to kill "all incurable charity patients, the aged who are a public care, wounded soldiers, all deformed children, the mentally afflicted," then we will no longer be living in our society. And it will have nothing to do with aid in dying.

In that society medical ethics will no longer exist in any meaningful way. We will no longer be worried about individual choice and assisted death because we will be murdering right and left, day and night. Our society, our culture will have vanished. Our Constitution will be gone. Is it sensible to think that aid in dying as allowed in Oregon will lead to the destruction of our common values? These argument are most certainly "overkill," so to speak.

3.   The Fears Are Misdirected

The opponents of aid in dying who predict terrible cultural shifts must also understand that their arguments are misdirected. It is not aid in dying which occasions their fears. There are other issues and events in medical ethics which are unrelated to aid in dying and which have more relevance to future fears of involuntary killing.

Here is a medical ethics discussion which veers away from aid in dying. It does so to explain further where we are in regard to death and dying issues and why aid in dying is not the end of life choice to be feared.

Let us join in the speculation. Let us predict that our societal climate will change and someone will propose that we take action to kill individuals who are minimally conscious or "vulnerable," or "disabled." And to make this more difficult we will not define "minimally conscious," "vulnerable," or "disabled." We will assume that the proposal is made in light of our limited resources and the desire to spend our available resources on patients who are "more of a benefit than a burden to society" and that "some lives are a nuisance and not worth living." How would that debate proceed? (Again, this discussion is simply intended to give further insight into the mistaken ethical reasoning of some opponents to aid in dying.)

One must understand what has already occurred in medical ethics relating to life, living, death and involuntary killing. Such an understanding demonstrates it will not be Oregon leading that imagined march to involuntary killings.

In that future debate we will argue about the concept of "personhood" and the differences between "life" and "living" and death. The arguments for involuntarily terminating the lives of those who are minimally conscious will be built on the cases of those who are permanently unconscious. It will not be founded on those who are conscious and making voluntary choices. Those other cases and concepts have already been raised and they cannot be avoided. They also significantly preceded the legalization of aid in dying in Oregon.

The meaning of life and death and when we must support one and may involuntarily hasten the other has been the subject of much attention and many cases in the past 50 years. Today we must worry about patients we did not have to worry about in the recent past. We did not have the medical knowledge and technology to keep many patients alive and they simply died. But because of our advances in medical science we can now maintain the physical body of an individual long after the loss of significant brain activity. We have been forced to make decisions we never had to make before.

If a feared proposal to eliminate the vulnerable should arise in the future what will be argued are issues similar to those involved in the 2013 California case of Jahi McMath and the 2005 Florida case of Terri Schiavo. These are patients who are either "brain dead" or in a persistent vegetative state.

Jahi and Brain Death

Jahi McMath can represent those patients who suffer a total cessation of brain function.

Jahi was a bright and energetic thirteen year old girl in Oakland, California, who underwent surgery in 2013 to treat a sleep apnea condition. After surgery something went terribly wrong and Jahi began to bleed profusely and went into cardiac arrest. Several days later she was determined to be "brain dead." Court proceedings ensued and eventually ended with a ruling that the hospital could remove all support. Although determined to be dead in accordance with California law, Jahi's family insisted that she remain on support. The family removed her body from the hospital to an undisclosed location. At the time of this writing, and as far as we know, her body is still being maintained with mechanical support. The ending is predictable.

We now have cultural definitions of death that include the concept of "brain death." In addition to irreversible cessation of circulatory and respiratory functions, we now declare a person dead if they have suffered "total cessation of brain activity, including the brain stem." Physicians may withdraw all medical support and notify the family of the death.

Many still argue against the concept of "brain death." They insist that to withdraw support of the body is wrong and amounts to killing a live human being. Those arguments have not prevailed.

Terri and the Permanently Unconscious

Next consider the tragic and well known Florida case of Terri Schiavo. Terri can represent our many current and future permanently unconscious patients. (Older readers may remember the similar 1976 New Jersey case of Karen Ann Quinlan.)

Terri was neither "brain dead" nor biologically dead. Her brain stem survived to allow her heart to beat and her lungs to breath. She was provided food and fluids through tubes. She even appeared to be awake at times. But she was permanently unconscious in a "persistent vegetative state." She would never regain a conscious existence.

In that infamous case her physical and mental conditions were debated. We questioned what she would have wanted and whether it was "futile" to continue providing medical support. We debated if it was ethical to withdraw support, including nutrition and liquids. (If only Terri had completed an advance directive telling us what to do in the event of such a tragic situation!)

In the end, and bypassing all of the nonsense that accompanied that unfortunate case, it was determined that it was proper to end medical support to bring about her biological death. In the end, her case was decided in accordance with prevailing ethical conclusions regarding permanently unconscious patients.

As with brain death, many thought that allowing the biological death of Terri was murder. And the same "culture of death" arguments were made. Those persons have not prevailed. We have resolved those cases and do not now think withdrawing all support from permanently unconscious persons is immoral and wrong.

Living Remains

How do we justify the decision to remove life support from these live human beings? How do we justify direct action to bring about their biological deaths? We justify such action because we do not believe a lack of brain function or being permanently unconscious amounts to "living." Yes, the body has life. There is biological life. But, the *person* is no longer living.

What does it mean to be a living human being? What does "living" mean? Doesn't "living" mean to have thoughts, plans, hopes, fears, relationships, joys, sorrows and all of those things that living human beings have. "Living" means to experience, to interact with the world and others, to think, to wish, feel, believe, love, and have desires. And, if an individual has lost all of those things, it is not that their life is not worth living, it is that *they* are not living.

When we bring about those deaths it is not because we do not respect life or no longer value life or because we trivialize the person's quality of life. It is because we understand that the living *person* is gone. Jahi and Terri were gone. We could not relate to their person and they could not relate to us. You are living in your home. Terri was in Florida but she was not living in Florida.

What we have in such cases are the living remains of persons who have died. We might more properly label it "living remains support" as "life support."

With cases of brain death and cases such as Terri it is the same understanding. These are not simply "persons with disabilities" or "cognitively disabled" patients. The physical condition of the body is of little concern. No matter the extent of physical disability or lack of mobility. Is the *person* still alive? Do they have thoughts and hopes and fears? Are Jahi and Terri *living*? An individual without those things is not a living person no matter how perfect the heart and limbs. An individual with those things is a living person to be treated with respect no matter how imperfect or disabled the physical body may be.

There is an alternative course of action for patients like Jahi and Terri. We can maintain their biological life for as long as possible. Karen Ann Quinlan was unconscious for nine years before death arrived. Terri for fifteen. Jahi? We can maintain permanently unconscious patients for ten, twenty or forty years. Should we be obligated in each and every case to go for a record?

We have sidestepped into this discussion of "brain death" and permanently unconscious patients because it can help us further understand why the fears of some are misdirected at aid in dying. In the extraordinarily unlikely event that their fears come to pass, the path to the involuntary killing of the old and vulnerable will lead from the involuntary deaths of the brain dead and permanently unconscious. The path will not lead from aid in dying. In fact, the path from aid in dying leads us in the opposite direction because it is built upon the voluntary choice of individuals.

4.   What is the Experience?

If aid in dying will lead us to any of the feared consequences then we should see some evidence this is occurring in Oregon and other states. After over sixteen years there should be some evidence that control is impossible or the "respect for human life" has begun to diminish.

If one has serious fears about aid in dying then one should seriously study what has been and is occurring in Oregon and other states. If one is not serious and simply wishes to advance arguments to oppose aid in dying, then the experience can be ignored or trivialized.

From the beginning the State of Oregon has published reports of the results of the Death With Dignity Act. Those reports are easily accessible on line. There is much interesting information in Oregon's history to demonstrate that the fears of some have not been realized. The report for 2013 shows consistency with previous years and evidences exactly what many predicted would be the effect of permitting aid in dying.

In 2013 prescriptions were written for 122 individuals and 71 deaths were reported. Of the 71 deaths, most were aged 65 or older with a median age of 71 years. Most were well-educated and had cancer. Most had some form of health care insurance. Two patients were referred for formal psychiatric or psychological evaluation. Nearly all died at home and most were enrolled in hospice care. (A significant benefit of permitting aid in dying in Oregon is that much more thought and effort is being given to end of life care and options for all patients.)

Because we knew what to worry about and how to design safeguards, none of the fears of opponents have come to pass. None.

Beyond these facts, what about the attitude of those living in Oregon? Is Oregon society facing "serious societal risks? Is there any evidence that the culture of Oregon more resembles a "culture of death" than the cultures of Texas or Florida? Let the social scientists continue their work. (Is it aid in dying or the increasing availability of guns with expanded permission to use them that will create a future "culture of death?")

5. Attack the Experience and the Proponents

Finally, you will hear arguments attacking both the experience and the proponents of aid in dying.

The worst enemy of those who oppose assisted death is our continuing experience. Further experience means we will have even more evidence that the predicted harms are not inevitable and can be avoided. Because this is true we see commentary attacking the experience in Oregon. We are not being given the full story. We are not being told the truth. Horror stories are being hushed up. Terrible things are happening. There is a massive conspiracy at work.

The fact is the citizens of Oregon, Washington and Vermont are no different than other Americans. They love life. They seek better and longer lives. They are concerned about unethical practices. They care about their family, friends and neighbors. They have also demonstrated that aid in dying can be permitted without the terrible harms predicted by some.

Proponents of aid in dying are also attacked. They have, of course, a hidden agenda. It is not individual freedom and the relief of suffering they seek. It is the eventual killing off of the old and vulnerable. They are fooling the rest of us into believing they care about the dying.

Such attacks often occur in the debates surrounding aid in dying. This is a failure to acknowledge that good people acting in good faith can have different views. It is simply that we are diverse. We have different feelings and beliefs. We have different understandings regarding life and death. Some see harmful consequences. Some see benefit.

We should approach each other in good faith in the attempt to resolve these important public policy questions.

Part Five

What Aid In Dying is Really About

We have discussed the desire of some dying individuals to hasten death. We have discussed feelings and beliefs and the role and limits of ethical inquiry. We have considered the role of the physician. We have discussed the fears of some and their dire predictions of the future. But what is aid in dying really about?

Aid In dying is about managing the deaths of the dying. No more. No less. Here is a straightforward explanation of what aid in dying is about.

Most of us know several things. We know death is the natural end to life. We know we are going to die. We know the modern dying process may be extraordinarily difficult and may be prolonged by medical knowledge and technology. We may even be "intubated and electrified with bizarre mechanical companions." We know that it can involve significant pain and/or suffering. While we hope for the best, we know "things could go wrong" and we may become one of the few that conclude that our continued dying is worse than our impending death.

Because we know these things we think several other things. We probably will not want to hasten our deaths but in the event the dying process does become unbearable, we would appreciate an additional option. The ability to request and receive the assistance of a physician in death seems to be a good additional option. We think this is a personal decision and we think we should have this option. We believe this is sensible. We think aid in dying can be managed with no more difficulty than many other aspects of life and medicine. Reasonable safeguards to prevent possible abuses are proper and can be fashioned as has been done in Oregon, Washington and Vermont. This is what aid in dying is about.

It is not about "suicide" and our individual religious and moral views concerning "suicide." The person is dying.

It is not about causing the deaths of those who are not dying. That is another subject altogether.

It is not about the desire of some to kill the vulnerable, the old, the disabled or any person who is not dying. Who is thinking that?

While it is that simple, we can offer a more complicated explanation of what assisted death is about. Many have. It is what theologians, philosophers and bioethicists love to do (including the author).

We can talk about the nature and meaning of human existence. We can wonder about life, death, man's relationship to God, and the moral significance of being old or in pain. We can debate the importance of control over death, the importance of suffering and disability, the nature of rights and obligations, ancient medical traditions, selfishness, the meaning of free choice, and on and on and on. Is aid in dying about those subtle and sophisticated theological and moral concepts? Well, yes. We can talk about those things and what they mean to us as individuals. But they fail to understand the concern and they miss the point.

Individual Choice and Timing

Aid in dying is not about whether we live or die. We are living. We will die. If you are dying, death will come soon or sooner. Aid in dying is about individual choice and timing. No more. No less.

This end of life choice is supported by well-established medical and social ethical principles which should apply to all dying patients.

We believe individuals may hasten death by refusing life saving medical care. We defend the choice to withdraw from treatment and die. We allow the dying to hurry death by refusing further food and drink. We will follow your advance directive and bring about your death if that is your wish. These are all instances where we emphasize the importance of individual choice in the timing of death.

Although aid in dying is also about individual choice and timing, it is forbidden in some states. Why? Because some are willing to use force to keep all of society in line with their religious beliefs. Because some allege a duty never to assist death (although that duty is bent beyond recognition in many ways every day). Because some see unsupported visions of terrible consequences and refuse to acknowledge our experience and ability to care for ourselves.

The Shift

A shift is occurring. It began in Oregon and it will continue. The shift involves all three of the objections to aid in dying.

The shift is a recognition that we are diverse in our feelings, beliefs and thinking. It is a recognition that we are uncertain regarding ultimate right and wrong in these matters. We understand that good people acting in good faith can disagree.

The shift is toward a greater appreciation for personal moral guidance and choice. We understand that we can live in peace and freedom with one another only if we tolerate the views and choices of others.

The shift is away from religious, moral and ethical bullies claiming the right to use force against those who disagree with them even though they cannot establish that their feelings, beliefs or ethical reasoning are superior.

The shift is an understanding that, even when we are dying, our physicians can assist us to the end, respecting our situation and desires. We also understand that neither patient nor physician must do anything. Aid in dying is permitted. It is not mandated.

The shift is an understanding that aid in dying does not create new risks that cannot be anticipated and avoided. Allowing the dying a choice and emphasizing the importance of individual freedom actually offers protection against those who might seek to cause involuntary deaths.

The shift is away from those who claim to see the future and predict that the worst of human nature will prevail. The experience in Oregon and Washington and newer states will continue to assure us that sensible ideas and the usual vigilance are protection enough.

The shift is not with our view of death. The people of Oregon, Washington and Vermont do not now love death, encourage death, and look for ways to expand killing. They wish for long and healthy lives as much as other human beings. They have as much care and compassion for the sick and dying as other Americans. They appreciate medical efforts to improve health and extend meaningful life and living.

At the same time, the shift *is* with our view of death. Some human beings fully understand that death is the natural and inevitable end to life. They have concluded that their earthly death is not the worst thing that can happen to them. A society that refuses to understand that death is the natural end to life and which insists that death is always a harm, always a danger, and must always be denied, is a society that fails to recognize the obvious.

This is what aid in dying is really about.

Part Six

The Ultimate Conclusion

The ultimate question is: Should aid in dying be permitted as a matter of public policy?

We are required to come together in good faith to discuss these important issues. We must work to understand each other and to appreciate certain truths.

We are diverse. We have different feelings and beliefs. We do not know the secrets of the universe in regard to what is ultimately right and wrong. We want to live in peace with our neighbors. We want to be free to make highly personal decisions which do not harm others. We are capable of creating sensible laws which provide reasonable safeguards.

These are the understandings that have convinced other states to follow the Oregon trail involving aid in dying.

While more can be said about everything, enough has been said. And while reason and experience support aid in dying, opponents will continue to rely upon fear. It is always difficult to overcome the forces of fear.

You may read and understand this entire discussion and still oppose aid in dying. You may be certain that you will never seek to hasten your own death. You may even attempt to convince others that they should not seek aid in dying.

If you are a priest, minister, rabbi or imam you may preach to your flock that aid in dying is a sin and to be avoided.

If you are a physician you may refuse to participate.

If you worry about the future you may remain vigilant to prevent your fears from becoming reality.

What no one can do, however, is justify the use of force against those who see things differently.

It cannot be shown that the choice of the dying individual is wrong. It cannot be shown that the assistance of a physician is wrong. It cannot be shown that aid in dying leads to terrible harms. There are no further reasons for prohibition.

The ultimate conclusion is: There are no ethical arguments which justify the criminalization of aid in dying in our secular, pluralistic society. None.

About the Author

Byron Chell is retired and lives in Eugene, Oregon.

His education and experience are in philosophy and law. He has spent much of the past 35 years considering and teaching bioethics and the issues surrounding death and dying. It is hoped that this analysis will clarify and correct much of the confusion and misrepresentation that yet surrounds aid in dying.

Questions, comments or criticisms are welcome at **theultimateargument.com**

Made in the USA
San Bernardino, CA
22 February 2015